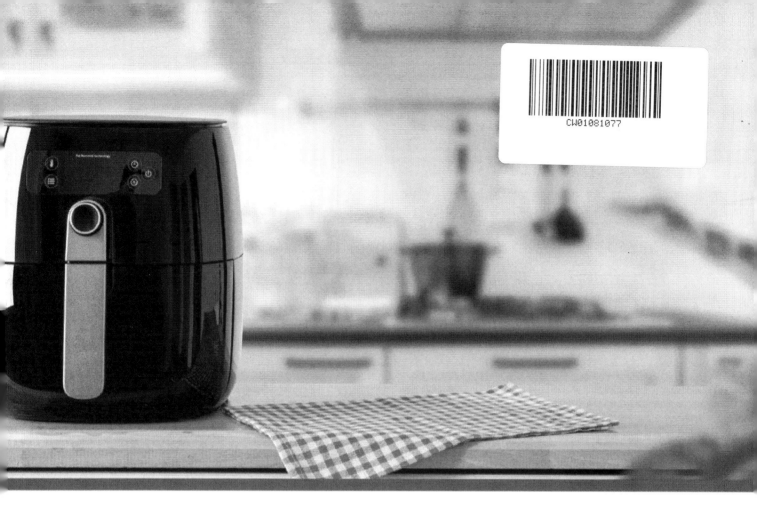

DIABETIC AIR FRYER COOKBOOK

The Ultimate Guide To Prepare Healthy Air Fryer Fried Dishes With Low Fat, Low Sugar, And Low Carb To Manage Type 1 And Type 2 Diabetes.

ERICA DIASON

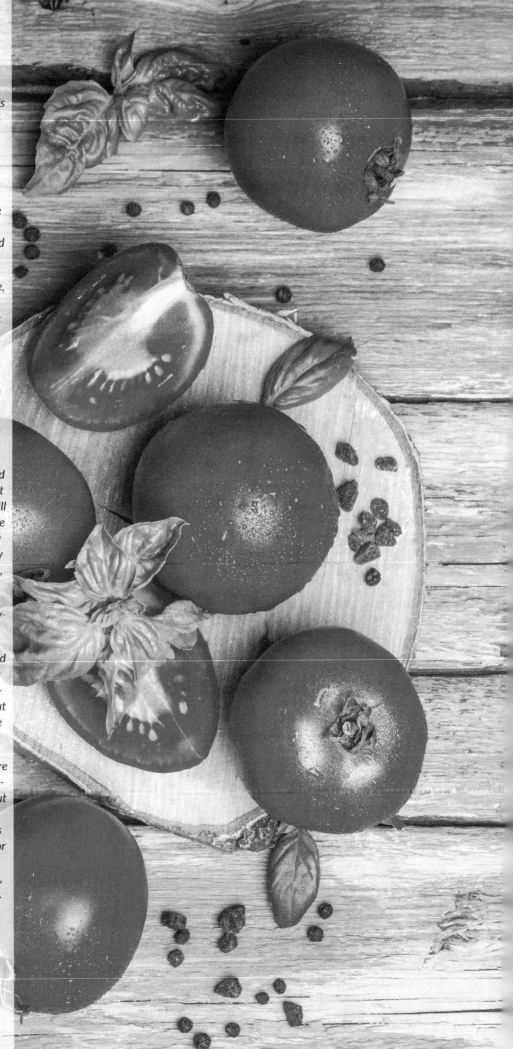

TABLE OF CONTENTS

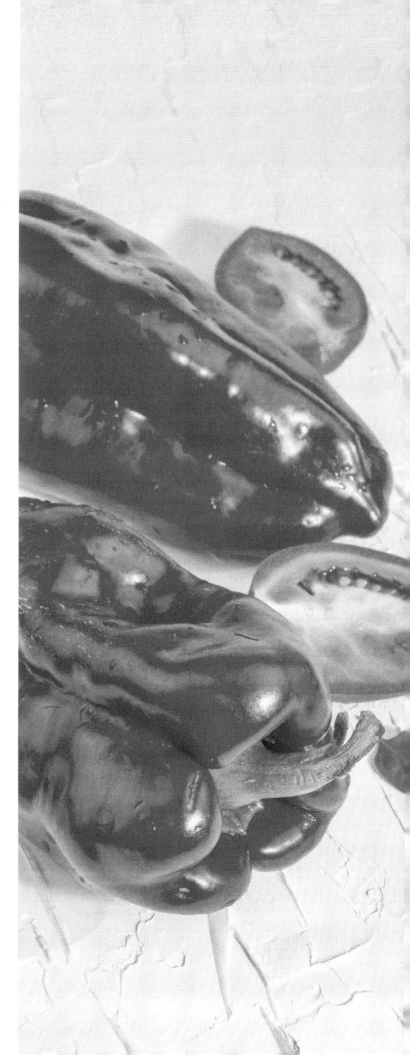

INTRODUCTION

Obesity is a medical condition when an individual has gained body fat too much, which can cause bad effects on their health. This varies from becoming overweight, where bone, muscle mass, fat, or body water growing to be the cause of the weight. A person is deemed obese if they weigh at least 20 pounds more than a healthy weight. For several different causes, obesity may occur, such as eating too many calories, contributing to an inactive lifestyle, and inadequate sleep. But irrespective of the cause, Obesity increases the risk of serious illnesses, including heart disease, type 2 diabetes, and high blood pressure.

There is a significant chance of having type 2 diabetes in obese individuals, which is often classified as adult-onset diabetes or insulin-resistant. This is a disorder when the amount of glucose in the blood is consistently high. In obese people, fat tissue cells could process more calories than they can consume. An inflammation activates a protein called cytokinesis caused by the tension in these cells by consuming too many nutrients. Cytokines, therefore, block insulin receptor signals, allowing the cells to become immune to insulin eventually. Insulin encourages glucose to be used by the cells for nutrition. Your body will be unable to turn the glucose into energy because your cells are immune to insulin, and you wind up with a consistently elevated blood glucose level.

Stress often induces inflammation of cells and may contribute to heart failure, in addition to reducing natural responses to insulin. Becoming obese or overweight raises the risk of having the prevalent type 2 diabetes; the body contains adequate insulin, yet the body's cells have become immune to insulin's action. The insides of human cells are strained by extra weight. The cell's membrane sends out a warning signal asking the cell to diminish the insulin cell surface receptors whenever the cells have more nutrients to absorb than they can accommodate. This represents insulin intolerance and persistently elevated sugar glucose in the blood, one of the clear diabetes indicators.

Diabetic patients are more likely to have severe heart complications, such as diabetic cardiomyopathy, coronary artery disease, heart failure, relative to individuals without diabetes. The heart needs to function particularly hard in obese or diabetic people by moving blood across the body as a consequence of the buildup of fatty substances all through the arteries. For people affected by obesity, particularly those with type 2 diabetes, weight reduction is an important approach. Moderate and consistent weight reduction, at least 5–10% weight reduction, will increase insulin activity, reduce the rate of fasting blood glucose, and decrease the need for certain drugs for diabetes.

To reverse diabetes symptoms, or at least to reduce the chances of getting diabetes, you must observe your lifestyle. An exercise, healthy diet, and behavior change program that will handle obesity effectively. These variables will significantly assist you with managing obesity and type 2 diabetes.

- Balance and healthy diet
- Physical exercise
- Medications

Physical Exercise is as necessary as medication, but an air fryer comes in handy when it comes to a healthy and balanced diet.

By regulating your diet and observing what you consume and how it affects your body, you can accomplish weight loss. You can now enjoy healthy fried foods. Although fried food goes together with healthy food, now it is possible to cook healthy food with an air fryer. Air frying is, on certain standards, easier than cooking in oil. It decreases calories by 70-80% and has a ton less fat.

This form of cooking may also minimize any of the other adverse consequences of oil frying. When you fry starchy foods, the product of this reaction creates the chemical acrylamide, which evidence ties to higher cancer risks. Air fryers offer the flavor, feel, and golden-brown color of oil-fried foods without all the calories. Air fryers are cooking devices that fry food by rotating heated air across the food. To achieve a comparable flavor and feel, air-fried foods are claimed to be safer and healthier than deep-fried foods since they need less oil.

Now, you can enjoy a healthier version of fast-fried food without worrying about the consequences.

Chapter 1.

DIABETES AND OBESITY

Diabetes is a stubborn condition that arises from two reasons when the pancreas cannot produce Insulin enough for body needs or whenever the Insulin it provides may not be utilized properly by the body. Insulin is a blood sugar-regulating hormone. Hyperglycemia, or high blood sugar, is a typical result of uncontrolled diabetes, causing significant harm to the body's structures, especially blood vessels and nerves over time. Diabetes mellitus is a category of illnesses that influence how the body uses glucose. Glucose is essential to your well-being. The cells that make up the muscles and tissues require a significant supply of glucose. It's the brain's primary power supply, too. The primary issue of diabetes varies based on the type of diabetes. And this can result in excessive sugar in the blood, no matter what kind of diabetes a person has. If there is too much sugar, it can lead to grave health issues. The insulin hormone transfers the sugar into the cells from the blood.

High levels of blood sugar may cause harm to your kidneys, eyes, organs, and nerves.

To understand what is the main reason for diabetes, you should know what the normal route of glucose consumption in the body is.

1. HOW GLUCOSE AND INSULIN WORK TOGETHER

The pancreas is an organ situated behind and below the stomach that produces Insulin. It is a hormone that regulates the level of sugar in the blood. Here is a step-by-step production in the bloodstream; insulin comes from the pancreases.

Then Insulin helps the sugar to go into the body cells.

Insulin reduces the level of sugar in the blood.

Now that the level of sugar drops in blood, it also causes the pancreas to secret less amount of Insulin.

- As blood sugar level drops in the body, it reduces insulin secretion from the pancreas.

2. TYPES OF DIABETES

A metabolic disorder that induces elevated blood sugar is diabetes mellitus, also known as diabetes. To be processed or used for nutrition, the hormone insulin transfers sugar from the blood in the cells. In diabetes, the body does not contain sufficient Insulin or does not utilize the Insulin it generates efficiently. Your brains, lungs, kidneys, and other organs may be affected by uncontrolled elevated blood sugar levels from diabetes.

There are different types of diabetes:

Type 1 Diabetes

A deficiency of the immune system, or an autoimmune disease, results in Type 1 diabetes, also called insulin-dependent diabetes or juvenile diabetes. In the pancreas, your immune system destroys the insulin-producing cells, killing the body's capacity to create Insulin. It's not clear what causes autoimmune disease and how to treat it effectively. You have to take Insulin to survive with Type 1 diabetes. As an infant or young adult, several individuals are diagnosed. Only 10% of people with diabetes have type 1 diabetes. Symptoms that the body shows on the onset of type 1 diabetes are polyuria (excessive excretion of urine), polydipsia (extreme thirst), sudden weight loss, constant hunger, fatigue, and vision changes. These changes can occur suddenly.

Type 2 Diabetes

Also known as adult-onset diabetes or non-insulin-dependent diabetes, it is caused by the body's inadequate insulin use. Type 2 diabetes is found in the majority of individuals with diabetes. The symptoms can be identical to those with type 1 diabetes. However, much less marked, as a consequence, when symptoms have already occurred, the condition can be detected after many years of diagnosis.

Type 2 diabetes happens when sugar starts adding up in your blood, and the body becomes resistant to Insulin. Type 2 diabetes is insulin resistance. Which ultimately leads to obesity. This in itself is a collection of different diseases. Older generations were more susceptible, but more and more young generations are now being affected. This is a product of bad health, not enough nutrition, and fitness patterns. Your pancreas avoids utilizing Insulin properly in type 2 diabetes. This creates complications with sugar that has to be taken out of the blood and placing it for energy in the cells. Finally, this will add to the need for insulin treatment.

Earlier stages, such as prediabetes, can be controlled successfully through food, exercise, and dynamic blood sugar control. This will also avoid the overall progression of type 2 diabetes. It is possible to monitor diabetes. In certain situations, if sufficient adjustments to the diet are created; on the contrary, the body will go into remission.

Gestational Diabetes

Hyperglycemia with blood glucose levels over average but below those diabetes levels is diagnosed with gestational diabetes. Gestational diabetes is identified via prenatal tests rather than by signs recorded—high blood sugar, which also occurs during gestation. Hormones produced by the placenta are Insulin-blocking, which is the main cause of this type of diabetes. You can manage gestational diabetes much of the time by food and exercise. Usually, it gets resolved after delivery. During pregnancy, gestational diabetes will raise the risk of complications. It will also increase the likelihood that both mothers and infants may experience type 2 diabetes later in life. This form of diabetes is caused by the placenta's production of insulin-blocking hormones.

3. THE CAUSES OF DIABETES

Causes of Type 1 Diabetes

Type 1 diabetes has an uncertain etiology. It's understood that the immune system targets and eradicates the cells (in the pancreas) that produce Insulin. The immune system usually destroys viruses or infectious bacteria. This leaves little or no insulin for the human body. Sugar keeps building up in the bloodstream instead of being transferred into the cells.

Type 1 diabetes is believed to be triggered by a mixture of hereditary susceptibility and the environment's variables, but it is still uncertain precisely what those variables are. It is not assumed that weight is a variable in type 1 diabetes. Type1 develops as the pancreas' beta cells that produce Insulin are targeted and killed by the body's immune system, the body's ability to combat infection. Scientists assume that type 1 diabetes is triggered by genetic makeup and environmental causes that could induce the condition.

Causes of Prediabetes and Type 2 Diabetes

Your cells can become immune to Insulin's effect in prediabetes, which can happen in type 2 diabetes, and the pancreas is not able to generate sufficient insulin to counteract this resistance. Sugar starts building up in your bloodstream instead of going to your cells, where it's required for fuel. Although genetic and environmental factors are believed to play a role in the development of type 2 diabetes, it is unclear why this occurs. The advancement of type 2 diabetes is closely related to being overweight, although not everybody with type 2 is obese. Several variables, including dietary conditions and genetic makeup, are responsible for the most prevalent type of diabetes.

Here are a few factors:

- **Insulin resistance**

Type 2 diabetes commonly progresses with insulin resistance, a disease in which Insulin is not handled well by the body, liver, and fat cells. As a consequence, to enable glucose to reach cells, the body requires more Insulin. The pancreas initially generates more Insulin to maintain the additional demand. The pancreas can't create enough insulin over time, and blood glucose levels increase.

- **Overweight, physical inactivity, and obesity**

When you are not regularly involved and are obese or overweight, you are much more prone to have type 2 diabetes. Often, excess weight induces insulin resistance, which is prominent in persons with type 2 diabetes. In which the fat stores of the body count a lot. Insulin tolerance, type 2 diabetes, heart, and blood artery dysfunction are attributed to excess belly fat.

- **Genes and family history**

A family history of diabetes in the family makes it more probable that gestational diabetes may occur in a mother, which means that genes play a part. In African Americans, Asians, American Indians, and Latinas, Hispanic, mutations can also justify why the disease happens more frequently.

Any genes can make you more susceptible to advance type 2 diabetes type 1 diabetes.

Genetic makeup can make a person more obese, which in turn leads to having type 2 diabetes.

Chapter 2.

HEALTHY LIVING AND AIR-FRYING

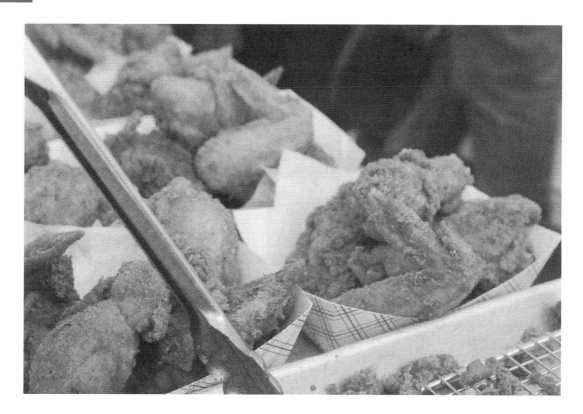

An air fryer is comparable to the oven in the way that it roasts and bakes. Still, the distinction is that the heating elements are situated only on top and supported by a strong, large fan, which results in very crisp food in no time. The air fryer utilizes spinning heated air to easily and uniformly cook food instead of using a pot of hot oil. In order to encourage the hot air to flow evenly around the meal, this is put in a metal basket (mesh) or a rack, producing the very same light golden, crispy crunch you get from frying in oil. It is an easy-to-use air fryer, cooks food faster than frying, and cleans up quickly. You can prepare a selection of healthy foods such as fruits, beef, seafood, poultry, and more, in addition to making beneficial variants of your favorite fried foods such as chips, onion rings, or French fries.

4. HOW AN AIR FRYER WORKS?

The air fryer is a convective heat oven with a revved-up countertop. Its small room enables cooking much quicker. A heating device and a fan are kept at the top of the device. Hot air flows through and around food put in a basket-type fryer. This fast circulation, just like deep frying, renders the food crisp. It's also super quick to clean up, and most systems include dishwasher-safe components.

5. COOKING IN AN AIR FRYER?

Air fryers are quick, and they're used to heat frozen foods or cook all kinds of fresh food, such as poultry, salmon, other seafood, pork chops, and vegetables, once you learn how it works. Since they are still so moist, most meats don't need additional oil:

Season them with salt and your favorite herbs and spices.

Be sure you adhere to dry seasonings; less moisture contributes to outcomes that are crispier.

Wait for the last few minutes of cooking, whether you choose to baste the beef with any sauce or barbecue sauce.

Lean meat cuts, or items containing minimal or no fat, need browning, and crisping needs a spray of oil. Before frying, clean the pork chops, boneless chicken breasts, and spray with a touch of oil. Due to the higher smoke point, vegetable oil or canola oil is generally preferred, which ensures that it can survive an air fryer's extreme heat.

Before air-fried, vegetables often need to be sprayed with oil. Sprinkle them with salt. Use less than you usually would use. The air-fried crispy bits carry a great deal of flavor. You will love fried baby potato halves, broccoli florets, and Brussels sprouts. They're so crisp. Everything tends to get sweeter with sweet potatoes, butternut squash, peppers, and green beans do not need long at all.

6. TIPS FOR COOKING IN AN AIR FRYER FOR BEGINNERS

Shake the basket: Make sure to open the fryer and move food around while they cook in the device's tray, compressing smaller foods such as French fries and chips. Toss them every 5–10 minutes for better performance.

Do not overcrowd the basket: Giving plenty of room to foods so that the air will efficiently circulate what gets you crispy outcomes.

Spray oil on the food: Make sure the food doesn't cling to the bowl. Gently brush foods with cooking spray.

Keep the food dry: To prevent splattering and excessive smoke, make sure food is dry before frying (even if you marinate it). In the same way, be sure to remove the grease from the bottom of the machine regularly while preparing high-fat items such as chicken wings.

Know other functions of air frying: The air fryer is not just for frying; it is also perfect for other healthier cooking methods, such as grilling, baking, and roasting.

Few other tips are:

Cut the food into equally sized parts for uniform cooking.

Distribute the food in one thin, even layer in the air fryer basket. If crowded the basket, food can be less crispy.

A tiny amount of oil would create the very same light, golden, crispy crust from frying. Using cooking spray or an oil mister to apply a thin, even coating oil to the food.

Air fryer is valuable for reheating foods, particularly with the crispy crust that you want.

7. BENEFITS OF USING AIR FRYER

- Easy cleanup
- Low-fat meals
- Less oil is needed

- Hot air cook's food evenly
- Weight loss
- Reduced cancer risk
- Diabetes management
- Improved memory
- Improved gut health

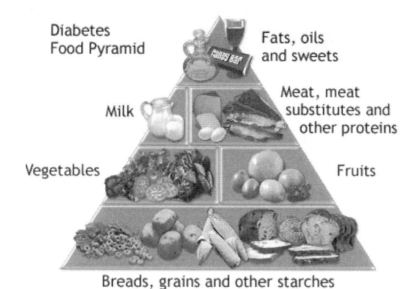

According to this food pyramid, you must consume a large portion of healthy vegetables and whole-grain starches, a balanced amount of healthy fats, and proteins with small amounts of nuts and oils.

8. HEALTHY LIVING AND HEALTHY EATING HABITS

To obtain optimal health benefits, it is necessary to use the right combination of numerous nutrients. Generally, a healthy diet includes the following classes of foods:

- Starchy foods such as potatoes, bread, pasta, and rice in smaller portions.
- Big portions of vegetables and fruits.
- Little amounts of dairy and milk foods.
- Protein foods include meat, fish, eggs.
- Protein (non-dairy), including beans, nuts, pulses, and tofu.
- The fifth food segment that you consume is fatty and sugary goods. Sugary and Fatty things can, though, make up just a limited portion of what you consume.
- Must eat salmon, sardines, and pilchards.
- Must eat dark green vegetables like broccoli and kale.
- Foods enriched in calcium, such as fruit juices and soya goods.
- Vitamin D allows the body to digest calcium, so try to go outdoors to receive vitamin D from the sun, have enough vitamin D-containing items, such as fortified cereal, fatty fish in the diet.
- It's necessary, substitute saturated fat with polyunsaturated fat.
- Consume at least five vegetable and fruit portions a day.
- Consume a minimum of two portions of fish each week (ideally fatty fish).
- Start consuming entire grains and nuts daily.
- Keep the sum of salt to very little, like 6 g a day.
- Restricted the consumption of alcohol.

Limit or Avoid the Following in Diet

Commercially manufactured or processed meats, or readymade foods that are high in trans fatty acids and salt.

Refined grains, such as dried cereals or white bread.

Sweetened sugary beverages.

High-calorie yet nutritionally weak foods, such as cookies, desserts, and crisps.

A Well-Balanced Diet Includes All the Following

You need the stamina to be productive during the day.

Nutrients you need to develop and restore help you remain balanced and powerful and help avoid diet-related diseases, such as diabetes and certain cancers.

You may also help sustain a healthier weight by staying busy and consuming a healthy, nutritious diet.

Deficiencies of some vital nutrients, such as vitamins C, A, B, and E, and selenium, zinc, and iron, can impair the immune system's parts.

You will reduce the chances of developing type 2 diabetes and better heart health and will make your teeth & bones by keeping a healthier weight and consuming a nutritious diet low in saturated fat and rich in fiber that is found in whole grains.

Eating a balanced diet in the proper amounts, coupled with exercise, will also help you lose weight, lower cholesterol and blood pressure levels, and reduce the chances of type 2 diabetes.

Here Is How Your Blood Glucose Level Should Look Like

Mg/DL	Fasting	After Eating	2-3 hours After Eating
Normal	80-100	170-200	120-140
Impaired Glucose	101-125	190-230	140-160
Diabetic	126 +	220-300	200 +

Chapter 3.

DIETARY REQUIREMENTS OF DIABETICS

When treating diabetes, nutrition is a key component that should be deliberated. A balanced meal plan will help you control your blood sugar levels and keep them in the target range, among other things. To effectively manage your blood sugar level, you should balance what you drink and eat.

What you eat, how much you eat, and your timing is crucial in managing your blood sugar levels. The answer to all this is what I will share with you here.

9. MACRONUTRIENTS

When talking about healthy living, we can't proceed without mentioning macronutrients. So what are they?

Macronutrients are also called macros. They are nutrients our body needs in large quantities to function properly. The nutrients provide your body with energy measured in kcals or calories. There are three types of macronutrients:

Carbohydrates

Carbohydrates supply energy to the body. They are broken down into glucose and monosaccharides. Carbohydrates are not equal; they are either simple or complex.

Simple carbohydrates: These comprise small molecules that are digested easily and are responsible for a rapid increase in glucose levels.

Complex carbohydrates: Unlike the simple ones, larger molecules are broken down into smaller molecules. They take time to digest and are slow in increasing blood sugar.

The rapid consumption of carbohydrates will increase plasma glucose levels, which is measured by a glycemic index. Eating carbohydrates with a high glycemic index can easily increase your blood sugar glucose. On the other hand, eating foods with a low glycemic load will slowly increase your plasma glucose level.

Protein

Protein supplies the body with amino acids; the functions of the brain, blood, nervous system, hair, and skin are all made up of amino acids. It's also in charge of carrying oxygen and other vital nutrients all over the body. When carbohydrates and glucose are not available, the body will reverse-process protein to have energy.

Your body can make 11 amino acids on its own and get the other nine that it can't make through diet.

There are two types of protein, animal-based, and plant-based. Examples of plant-based proteins are seeds, nuts, and grains. The most common sources of protein can be sourced from meat, seafood products, eggs, and dairy.

According to the USDA, the daily requirements of protein sources should be anywhere from 10% to 30% of your daily calories.

Fats

Generally, people see fat as bad and try to avoid it in their diet. However, dietary fat is important in your journey of maintaining your sugar level low. Good fats protect your organs, allow proper cell function, and are also important for insulin. In terms of caloric deprivation or starving, fat can be a source of energy.

While good fats are crucial for a healthy diet, bad fats can gradually contribute to obesity. To maintain a healthy weight, fats should be consumed in moderation. Let's quickly take a look at the different types of fats.

Saturated fats: Saturated fats come from dairy sources and meat. When at room temperature, they are solid and can be shelf-stable for a while.

Unsaturated fats: These are good fats that are either monounsaturated or polyunsaturated. They come from meat and some plant sources and are very beneficial. They are liquid under normal room temperature and remain so even after refrigeration. They have a shorter shelf life than saturated fats.

Trans Fats: These are polyunsaturated fats that change from liquid to solid form and are extremely unhealthy for you. They are used in processed food, fast food, cakes, cookies, and any other food that contains hydrogenated fats.

10. OTHER ESSENTIAL NUTRIENTS

Besides macros, which provide your body with nutrients, there are other essential nutrients you need to consider. These nutrients are also essential and need to be included in your diet.

Vitamin D

Vitamin D is a little deliberated fat-soluble hormone that provides many benefits. It helps in maintaining joints, bones, teeth and boosts the immune system. Examples of foods you can get the vitamin from include nuts, eggs, seeds, butter, and oily fish.

Additionally, by exposing yourself to the sun for 30 minutes daily, you encourage your vitamin D production and reduce your risk for diabetes.

Magnesium

This is a must-have nutrient in your diet. Research has suggested that people with Type 2 diabetes are more likely to have a deficiency in magnesium. Intracellular magnesium is responsible for vascular tone, regulating insulin's actions, and insulin-mediated glucose uptake. So, being deficient in magnesium isn't good, as it can worsen insulin resistance. Correcting a deficiency in magnesium will greatly help you manage your condition better.

Sodium

The function of sodium in the body is to transmit nerve pulses and control the electric charge both inside and outside your cells. When we eat mostly processed foods, we are most likely to consume more sodium than we want. Even though a high sodium intake is bad, a low intake can affect insulin resistance and cause cardiovascular disease.

The American Dietary Guidelines suggested that a daily intake of 2,300 milligrams shouldn't be exceeded. If you can, limit it to 1,500 milligrams; the lesser, the better.

11. Recommended Nutrients for Diabetics

Nutrition is a crucial aspect that needs to be deliberated when treating diabetes. What goes into your system is part of what determines your blood sugar level. To maintain a proper blood sugar level, you need to pay attention to what you eat. Therefore, I will be sharing with you the recommended nutrients for diabetes. These are healthy foods you should stock your kitchen with.

Vegetables

- Carrots
- Broccoli
- Tomatoes
- Green peas
- Green pepper

Fruits

- Berries (strawberries, blueberries, blackberries)
- Oranges
- Citrus
- Apples
- Grapes

Grains (whole grains)

- Oats
- Quinoa
- Barley
- Cornmeal
- Brown rice

Dairy: low-fat

- Yogurt
- Milk
- Cheese
- Almond milk, soy milk

Protein

- Turkey or chicken without skin
- Lean meat
- Eggs
- Fish
- Nuts
- Split peas
- Chickpeas
- Dried beans
- Meat substitutes (tofu)

The foods you can eat are not limited to my suggestions above. There are other healthy foods you can eat. Instead of stick margarine, shortening, and lard, make use of oils when cooking. Also, make sure you include foods with heart-healthy fats in your diet. Some of these include avocado, olive oil, canola, nuts and seeds, tuna, salmon, and mackerel.

Each nutrient has its specific roles in the body. Since you are managing a health condition, you need to balance them to avoid loading yourself up with excess carbs. A diabetic diet will help you figure out how to balance nutrients and make healthy choices.

12. WATCH WHAT YOU EAT

Watching what you eat is one of the things to do when controlling your blood sugar. The starches and sugars in your food significantly impact your body; this makes it very important to know what you are eating. To support this, there are some steps to take, and I have highlighted them below.

13. LEARN PORTION CONTROL

Portion control entails choosing a healthy size of certain foods. To effectively control your blood sugar, you need to be in control of the food you eat. Portion control can help you lose weight, digest food easily, stay energized, and reduce the intake of problematic foods. According to the (ADA) American Diabetes Association, your plate should have a lesser portion of starch and lean meats and a bigger portion of non-starchy vegetables.

14. LIMIT SOME FOODS AND DRINKS

Below are some foods and drinks you should limit to support your healthy eating journey.

- Foods high in sodium
- Sweets (ice cream, baked goods, and candy)
- Fried foods high in trans-fat and saturated fat
- Beverages with added sugar (soda, energy drinks, and juice)

I would advise you to drink water instead of drinking sweetened beverages. Also, consider using a sugar substitute for your food. Examples of healthy sugar substitutes include tagatose, stevia, neotame, and acesulfame potassium. Avoid aspartame and sucralose, which are not healthy.

If you can avoid drinking alcohol, please do. However, if you must drink, it should be in moderate quantities. Men shouldn't drink more than two drinks, and women shouldn't go beyond one drink. Alcohol can make your blood sugar level low or too high; it's best to be avoided. Also, avoid carb-rich drinks, like wine and beer

Chapter 4.

APPETIZER AND SIDES RECIPES

1. GARLIC KALE CHIPS

Preparation Time: 6–7 minutes

Cooking Time: 5 minutes

Servings: 2

Ingredients:

» 1 tbsp. yeast flakes
» Sea salt to taste
» 4 cups packed kale
» 2 tbsp. olive oil
» 1 tsp. garlic, minced
» 1/2 cup ranch seasoning pieces

Directions:

1. In a bowl, place the oil, kale, garlic, and ranch seasoning pieces. Add the yeast and mix well. Dump the coated kale into an air fryer basket and cook at 375°F for 5 minutes.
2. Shake after 3 minutes and serve.

Nutrition:

» Calories: 50
» Total Fat: 1.9 g
» Carbs: 10 g
» Protein: 46 g

2. GARLIC SALMON BALLS

Preparation Time: 6–7 minutes

Cooking Time: 10 minutes

Servings: 2

Ingredients:

» 6 oz. tinned salmon
» 1 large egg
» 3 tbsp. olive oil
» 5 tbsp. wheat germ
» 1/2 tsp. garlic powder
» 1 tbsp. dill, fresh, chopped
» 4 tbsp. spring onion, diced
» 4 tbsp. celery, diced

Directions:

1. Preheat your air fryer to 370°F. In a large bowl, mix the salmon, egg, celery, onion, dill, and garlic.
2. Shape the mixture into golf ball size balls and roll them in the wheat germ. In a minor pan, warm olive oil over medium-low heat. Add the salmon balls and slowly flatten them. Handover them to your air fryer and cook for 10 minutes.

Nutrition:

» Calories: 219
» Total Fat: 7.7 g
» Carbs: 14.8 g
» Protein: 23.1 g

3. ONION RINGS

Preparation Time: 7 minutes

Cooking Time: 10 minutes

Servings: 3

Ingredients:

- » 1 onion, cut into slices, then separate into rings
- » 1 ½ cup almond flour
- » 3/4 cup pork rinds
- » 1 cup milk
- » 1 egg
- » 1 tbsp. baking powder
- » 1/2 tsp. salt

Directions:

1. Preheat your air fryer for 10 minutes. Cut onion into slices, then separate into rings. In a container, supplement the flour, baking powder, and salt.
2. Whisk the eggs and the milk, then combines with flour. Gently dip the floured onion rings into the batter to coat them.
3. Spread the pork rinds on a plate and dredge the rings in the crumbs. Abode the onion rings in your air fryer and cook for 10 minutes at 360°F.

Nutrition:

- » Calories: 304
- » Total Fat: 18g
- » Carbs: 31g
- » Protein: 38g

4. CRISPY EGGPLANT FRIES

Preparation Time: 7 minutes

Cooking Time: 12 minutes

Servings: 3

Ingredients:

- » 2 eggplants
- » 1/4 cup olive oil
- » 1/4 cup almond flour
- » 1/2 cup water

Directions:

1. Preheat your air fryer to 390°F. Cut the eggplants into ½-inch slices. In a mixing bowl, mix the flour, olive oil, water, and eggplants.
2. Slowly coat the eggplants. Add eggplants to the air fryer and cook for 12 minutes. Serve with yogurt or tomato sauce.

Nutrition:

- » Calories: 103
- » Total Fat: 7.3 g
- » Carbs: 12.3 g
- » Protein: 1.9 g

5. CHARRED BELL PEPPERS

Preparation Time: 7 minutes

Cooking Time: 4 minutes

Servings: 3

Ingredients:

- 20 bell peppers, sliced and seeded
- 1 tsp. olive oil
- 1 pinch sea salt
- 1 lemon
- Pepper

Directions:

1. Preheat your air fryer to 390°F. Sprinkle the peppers with oil and salt. Cook the peppers in the air fryer for 4 minutes.
2. Place peppers in a large bowl, and squeeze lemon juice over the top. Season with salt and pepper.

Nutrition:

- Calories: 30
- Total Fat: 0.25 g
- Carbs: 6.91 g
- Protein: 1.28 g

6. GARLIC TOMATOES

Preparation Time: 7 minutes

Cooking Time: 15 minutes

Servings: 4

Ingredients:

- 3 tbsp. vinegar
- 1/2 tsp. thyme, dried
- 4 tomatoes
- 1 tbsp. olive oil
- Salt and black pepper to taste
- 1 garlic clove, minced

Directions:

1. Preheat your air fryer to 390°F. Scratch the tomatoes into halves and remove the seeds. Please place them in a big bowl and toss them with oil, salt, pepper, garlic, and thyme.
2. Place them into the air fryer and cook for 15 minutes. Drizzle with vinegar and serve.

Nutrition:

» Calories: 28.9
» Total Fat: 2.4 g
» Carbs: 2.0 g
» Protein: 0.4 g

7. MUSHROOM STEW

Preparation Time: 7 minutes

Cooking Time: 1 hour 22 minutes

Servings: 3

Ingredients:

- » 1 lb. chicken, cubed, boneless, skinless
- » 2 tbsp. canola oil
- » 1 lb. fresh mushrooms, sliced
- » 1 tbsp. thyme, dried
- » 1/4 cup water
- » 2 tbsp. tomato paste
- » 4 garlic cloves, minced
- » 1 cup green peppers, sliced
- » 3 cups zucchini, diced
- » 1 large onion, diced
- » 1 tbsp. basil
- » 1 tbsp. marjoram
- » 1 tbsp. oregano

Directions:

1. Cut the chicken into cubes. Position them in the air fryer basket and pour olive oil over them. Add mushrooms, zucchini, onion, and green pepper. Mix and add garlic, cook for 2 minutes, then add tomato paste, water, and seasonings.
2. Lock the air fryer and cook the stew for 50 minutes. Set the heat to 340°F and cook for an additional 20 minutes.
3. Remove from air fryer and transfer into a large pan. Empty in a bit of water and simmer for 10 minutes.

Nutrition:

- » Calories: 53
- » Total Fat: 3.3 g
- » Carbs: 4.9 g
- » Protein: 2.3 g

8. CHEESE & ONION NUGGETS

Preparation Time: 7 minutes

Cooking Time: 12 minutes

Servings: 4

Ingredients:

- » 7 oz. Edam cheese, grated
- » 2 spring onions, diced
- » 1 egg, beaten
- » 1 tbsp. coconut oil
- » 1 tbsp. thyme, dried
- » Salt and pepper to taste

Directions:

1. Mix the onion, cheese, coconut oil, salt, pepper, thyme in a bowl. Make 8 small balls and place the cheese in the center.
2. Place in the fridge for about an hour. With a pastry brush, carefully brush the beaten egg over the nuggets. Cook for 12 minutes in the air fryer at 350°F.

Nutrition:

- » Calories: 227
- » Total Fat: 17.3 g
- » Carbs: 4.5 g
- » Protein: 14.2 g

9. SPICED NUTS

Preparation Time: 7 minutes

Cooking Time: 25 minutes

Servings: 3

Ingredients:

- » 1 cup almonds
- » 1 cup pecan halves
- » 1 cup cashews
- » 1 egg white, beaten
- » 1/2 tsp. cinnamon, ground
- » Pinch cayenne pepper
- » 1/4 tsp. cloves, ground
- » Pinch salt

Directions:

1. Combine the egg white with spices. Preheat your air fryer to 300°F.
2. Toss the nuts in the spiced mixture. Cook for 25 minutes, stirring several times throughout cooking time.

Nutrition:

- » Calories: 88.4
- » Total Fat: 7.6 g
- » Carbs: 3.9 g
- » Protein: 2.5 g

10. KETO FRENCH FRIES

Preparation Time: 7 minutes

Cooking Time: 20 minutes

Servings: 4

Ingredients:

- » 1 large rutabaga, peeled, cut into spears about ¼-inch wide
- » Salt and pepper to taste
- » 1/2 tsp. paprika
- » 2 tbsp. coconut oil

Directions:

1. Preheat your air fryer to 450°F. Mix the oil, paprika, salt, and pepper.
2. Pour the oil mixture over the rutabaga fries, making sure all pieces are well coated. Cook in the air fryer for 20 minutes or until crispy.

Nutrition:

- » Calories: 113
- » Total Fat: 7.2 g
- » Carbs: 12.5 g
- » Protein: 1.9 g

11. FRIED GARLIC GREEN TOMATOES

Preparation Time: 7 minutes

Cooking Time: 12 minutes

Servings: 2

Ingredients:

- » 3 green tomatoes, sliced
- » 1/2 cup almond flour
- » 2 eggs, beaten
- » Salt and pepper to taste
- » 1 tsp. garlic, minced

Directions:

1. Season the tomatoes with salt, garlic, and pepper. Preheat your air fryer to 400°F. Dip the tomatoes first in flour then in the egg mixture.
2. Spray the tomato rounds with olive oil and place them in the air fryer basket. Cook for 8 minutes, then flip over and cook for additional 4 minutes. Serve with zero-carb mayonnaise.

Nutrition:

- » Calories: 123
- » Total Fat: 3.9 g
- » Carbs: 16 g
- » Protein: 8.4 g

12. GARLIC CAULIFLOWER TOTS

Preparation Time: 7 minutes

Cooking Time: 20 minutes

Servings: 4

Ingredients:

- » 1 crown cauliflower, chopped in a food processor
- » 1/2 cup parmesan cheese, grated
- » Salt and pepper to taste
- » 1/4 cup almond flour
- » 2 eggs
- » 1 tsp. garlic, minced

Directions:

1. Mix all the ingredients. Shape into tots and spray with olive oil. Preheat your air fryer to 400°F.
2. Cook for 10 minutes on each side.

Nutrition:

- » Calories: 18
- » Total Fat: 0.6 g
- » Carbs: 1.3 g
- » Protein: 1.8 g

Chapter 5.
POULTRY RECIPES

13. WARM CHICKEN AND SPINACH SALAD

Preparation Time: 10 minutes

Cooking Time: 16-20 minutes

Servings: 4

Ingredients:

- » 3 (5 oz.) low-sodium boneless, skinless chicken breasts, cut into 1-inch cubes
- » 5 tsp. olive oil
- » 1/2 tsp. dried thyme
- » 1 medium red onion, sliced
- » 1 red bell pepper, sliced
- » 1 small zucchini, cut into strips
- » 3 tbsp. freshly squeezed lemon juice
- » 6 cups fresh baby spinach

Directions:

1. In a huge bowl, blend the chicken with olive oil and thyme. Toss to coat. Transfer to a medium metal bowl and roast for 8 minutes in the air fryer.
2. Add the red onion, red bell pepper, and zucchini. Roast for 8 to 12 more minutes, stirring once during cooking, or until the chicken grasps an inner temperature of 165°F on a meat thermometer.
3. Remove the bowl from the air fryer and stir in the lemon juice.
4. Lay the spinach in a serving bowl and top with the chicken mixture. Toss to combine and serve immediately.

Nutrition:

- Calories: 214
- Fat: 7 g (29% of calories from fat)
- Saturated Fat: 1 g
- Protein: 28 g
- Carbs: 7 g
- Sodium: 116 mg
- Fiber: 2 g

14. DUO CRISP CHICKEN WINGS

Preparation Time: 10 minutes

Cooking Time: 18 minutes

Servings: 4

Ingredients:

- » 12 chicken vignettes
- » 1/2 cup chicken broth
- » Salt and black pepper to taste
- » 1/4 cup melted butter

Directions:

1. Set a metal rack in the air fryer oven and pour broth into it.
2. Place the vignettes on the metal rack.
3. Select 8 minutes of cooking time, then press "Start."
4. Once the air fryer oven beeps, transfer the cooked vignettes to a plate.
5. Empty the pot and set an air fryer basket in the oven.
6. Toss the vignettes with butter and seasoning.
7. Spread the seasoned vignettes in the air fryer basket.
8. Hit the "Air Fryer Button," then set the time to 10 minutes.
9. Serve and Enjoy

Nutrition:

- Calories 246
- Total Fat 18.9g
- Saturated Fat 7g
- Cholesterol 115mg
- Sodium 149mg
- Total Carbs: 0 g
- Dietary Fiber: 0 g
- Total Sugars: 0 g
- Protein: 20.2 g

15. AIR FRYER TERIYAKI HEN DRUMSTICKS

Preparation Time: 30 minutes

Cooking Time: 20 minutes

Servings: 4

Ingredients:

- » 6 poultry drumsticks
- » 1 mug teriyaki sauce

Directions:

1. Mix drumsticks with teriyaki sauce in a zip-lock bag. Let the sauce rest for half an hour.
2. Preheat your air fryer to 360°F.
3. Abode the drumsticks in one layer in the air fryer basket and cook for 20 minutes. Shake the basket pair times through food preparation.
4. Garnish with sesame seeds and sliced onions

Nutrition:

- Calories: 163
- Carbs: 7 g
- Protein: 16 g
- Fat: 7 g

16. CHICKEN PIE

Preparation Time: 10 minutes

Cooking Time: 17 minutes

Servings: 3

Ingredients:

- » 2 tbsp. olive oil
- » 1 pound chicken breast cubed
- » 1 tbsp. garlic powder
- » 1 tbsp. thyme
- » 1 tbsp. pepper
- » 1 cup chicken broth
- » 12 oz. bag frozen mixed vegetables
- » 4 large potatoes cubed
- » 10 oz. can chicken soup cream
- » 1 cup heavy cream

Directions:

1. Add chicken and olive oil to the air fryer.
2. Saute chicken for 5 minutes, then stirs in spices.
3. Pour in the broth along with vegetables and cream of chicken soup.
4. Select 10 minutes of cooking time, then press "Start."
5. Once the air fryer oven beeps, stir in cream and cook for 2 minutes.
6. Enjoy!

Nutrition:

- Calories 568
- Total Fat 31.1 g
- Saturated Fat: 9.1 g
- Cholesterol: 95 mg
- Sodium: 1111 mg
- Total Carbs: 50.8 g
- Dietary Fiber: 3.9 g
- Total Sugars: 18.8 g
- Protein: 23.4 g

17. CHICKEN CASSEROLE

Preparation Time: 10 minutes

Cooking Time: 9 minutes

Servings: 4

Ingredients:

- » 12 oz. bag egg noodles
- » 1/2 large onion
- » 1/2 cup chopped carrots
- » 1/4 cup frozen peas
- » 1/4 cup frozen broccoli pieces
- » 2 stalks celery chopped
- » 5 cups chicken broth
- » 1 tsp. garlic powder
- » Salt and pepper to taste
- » 1 cup cheddar cheese, shredded
- » 1 package French's onions
- » 1/4 cup sour cream
- » 1 can chicken cream and mushroom soup

Directions:

1. Add chicken broth, black pepper, salt, garlic powder, vegetables, and egg noodles to the air fryer oven.
2. Select 4 minutes of cooking time, then press "Start."
3. Once the air fryer oven beeps, stir in cheese, 1/3 of French's onions, a can of soup, and sour cream.
4. Mix well and spread the remaining onion on top.
5. Place in the air fryer and hit the "Air Fryer Button" and select 5 minutes of cooking time, then press "Start."
6. Serve and Enjoy.

Nutrition:

- Calories: 494
- Total Fat: 19.1 g
- Saturated Fat: 9.6 g
- Cholesterol: 142 mg
- Sodium: 1233 mg
- Total Carbs: 29 g
- Dietary Fiber: 2.6 g
- Total Sugars: 3.7 g
- Protein: 48.9 g

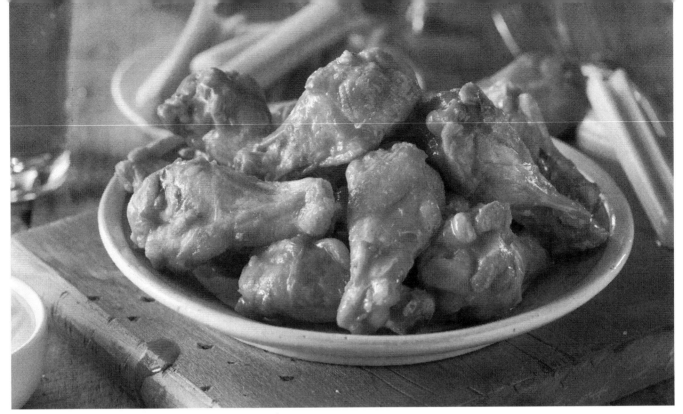

18. RANCH CHICKEN WINGS

Preparation Time: 10 minutes

Cooking Time: 35 minutes

Servings: 3

Ingredients:

- » 12 chicken wings
- » 1 tbsp. olive oil
- » 1 cup chicken broth
- » 1/4 cup butter
- » 1/2 cup red hot sauce
- » 1/4 tsp. Worcestershire sauce
- » 1 tbsp. white vinegar
- » 1/4 tsp. cayenne pepper
- » 1/8 tsp. garlic powder
- » Seasoned salt to taste
- » Black pepper
- » Ranch dressing for dipping
- » Celery to garnish

Directions:

1. Set the air fryer basket and pour the broth in it.
2. Spread the chicken wings in the basket.
3. Select 10 minutes of cooking time, then press "Start."
4. Meanwhile, for the sauce preparation, add butter, vinegar, cayenne pepper, garlic powder, Worcestershire sauce, and spicy sauce in a small saucepan.
5. Stir and cook this sauce for 5 minutes on medium heat until it thickens.
6. Once the air fryer oven beeps, remove the wings and empty the air fryer.
7. Toss the wings with oil, salt, and black pepper.
8. Set the air fryer basket in the oven and arrange the wings in it.
9. Hit the "Air Fryer Button" and select 20 minutes of cooking time, then press "Start."
10. Once the air fryer oven beeps, transfer the wings to the sauce and mix well. Serve.

Nutrition:

- Calories: 414
- Total Fat: 31.6 g
- Saturated Fat: 11 g
- Cholesterol: 98 mg
- Sodium: 568 mg
- Total Carbs: 11.2 g
- Dietary Fiber: 0.3 g
- Total Sugars: 0.2 g
- Protein: 20.4 g

19. CHICKEN MAC AND CHEESE

Preparation Time: 10 minutes

Cooking Time: 9 minutes

Servings: 4

Ingredients:

» 2 ½ cups macaroni
» 2 cups chicken stock
» 1 cup cooked chicken, shredded
» 1 ¼ cup heavy cream
» 8 tbsp. butter
» 1 bag Ritz crackers

Directions:

1. Add chicken stock, heavy cream, chicken, 4 tablespoons butter, and macaroni to the air fryer.
2. Select 4 minutes of cooking time, then press "Start."
3. Crush the crackers and mix them well with 4 tablespoons of melted butter.
4. Hit the "Air Fryer Button" again, select 5 minutes of cooking time adding crackers, then press "Start."
5. Once the air fryer oven beeps, serve.

Nutrition:

- Calories: 611
- Total Fat: 43.6 g
- Saturated Fat: 26.8g
- Cholesterol: 147 mg
- Sodium: 739 mg
- Total Carbs: 29.5 g
- Dietary Fiber: 1.2 g
- Total Sugars: 1.7 g
- Protein: 25.4 g

20. BACON-WRAPPED CHICKEN

Preparation Time: 10 minutes

Cooking Time: 24 minutes

Servings: 4

Ingredients:

» 1/4 cup maple syrup
» 1 tsp. ground black pepper
» 1 tsp. Dijon mustard
» 1/4 tsp. garlic powder
» 1/8 tsp. kosher salt
» 4 (6 oz.) skinless, boneless chicken breasts
» 8 slices bacon

Directions:

1. Whisk maple syrup with salt, garlic powder, mustard, and black pepper in a small bowl.
2. Rub the chicken with salt and black pepper, and wrap each chicken breast with 2 slices of bacon.
3. Place the wrapped chicken in the Air fryer baking pan.
4. Brush the wrapped chicken with maple syrup mixture.
5. Select 25 cooking times, then press "Start."
6. Serve.

Nutrition:

- Calories: 441
- Total Fat: 18.3 g
- Saturated Fat: 5.2 g
- Cholesterol: 141 mg
- Sodium: 1081 mg
- Total Carbs: 14 g
- Dietary Fiber: 0.1 g
- Total Sugars: 11.8 g
- Protein: 53.6 g

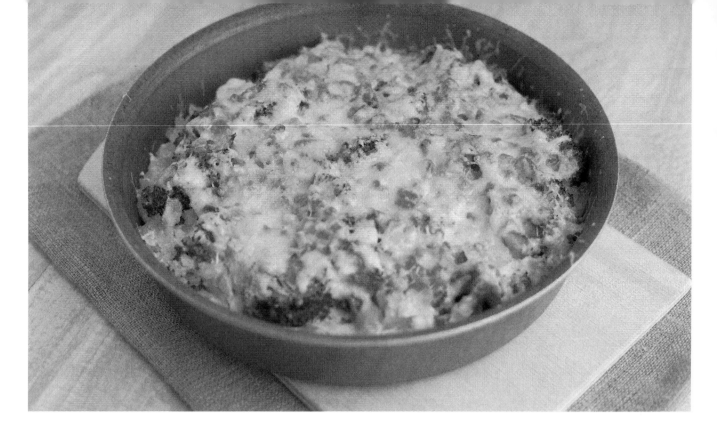

21. BROCCOLI CHICKEN CASSEROLE

Preparation time: 10 minutes

Preparation time: 22 minutes

Servings: 4

Ingredients:

- » 1 ½ lb. chicken, cubed
- » 2 tsp. chopped garlic
- » 2 tbsp. butter
- » 1 ½ cup chicken broth
- » 1 ½ cup long-grain rice
- » 1 (10.75 oz.) can chicken soup cream
- » 2 cups broccoli florets
- » 1 cup crushed Ritz cracker
- » 2 tbsp. melted butter
- » 2 cups shredded cheddar cheese
- » 1 cup water

Directions:

1. Swell 1 cup of water into the air fryer and place a basket in it.
2. Place the broccoli in the basket evenly.
3. Select 1 minute of cooking time, then press "Start."
4. Once the air fryer oven beeps, remove the broccoli and empty the air fryer.
5. Then add 2 tablespoons of butter.
6. Toss in chicken and stir cook for 5 minutes, then add garlic and saute for 30 seconds.
7. Stir in rice, chicken broth, and cream of chicken soup.
8. Select 12 minutes of cooking time, then press "Start."
9. Add cheese and broccoli once the air fryer oven beeps, then mix well gently.
10. Toss the cracker with 2 tablespoons butter in a bowl and spread over the pot's chicken.
11. Hit the "Air Fryer Button" and select 4 minutes of cooking time, then press "Start."
12. Once the air fryer beeps, serve.

Nutrition:

- Calories: 609
- Total Fat: 24.4 g
- Saturated: Fat 12.6g
- Cholesterol: 142 mg
- Sodium: 924mg

- Total Carbs: 45.5 g
- Dietary Fiber: 1.4 g
- Total Sugars: 1.6 g
- Protein: 49.2 g

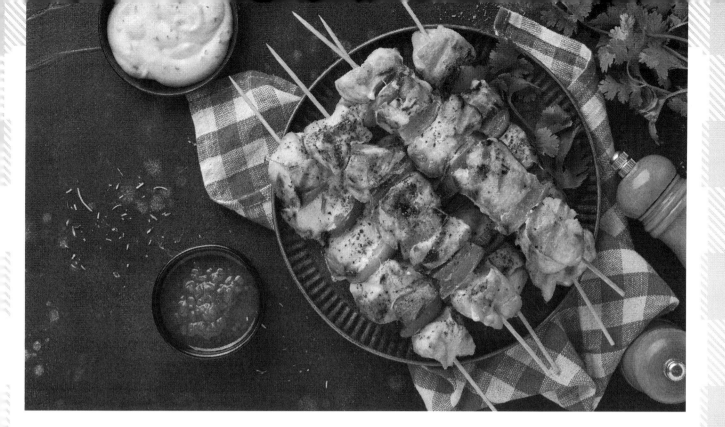

22. CHICKEN TIKKA KEBAB

Preparation Time: 10 minutes

Cooking Time: 17 minutes

Servings: 4

Ingredients:

» 1 lb. chicken thighs boneless skinless, cubed
» 1 tbsp. oil
» 1/2 cup red onion, cubed
» 1/2 cup green bell pepper, cubed
» 1/2 cup red bell pepper, cubed
» Lime wedges and Onion rounds to garnish

For marinade:

» 1/2 cup yogurt Greek
» 3/4 tbsp. ginger, grated
» 3/4 tbsp. garlic, minced
» 1 tbsp. lime juice
» 2 tsp. red chili powder mild
» 1/2 tsp. ground turmeric
» 1 tsp. garam masala
» 1 tsp. coriander powder
» 1/2 tbsp. dried fenugreek leaves
» 1 tsp. salt

Directions:

1. Preparation of the marinade by mixing yogurt with all its ingredients in a bowl.
2. Fold in chicken, then mix well to coat and refrigerate for 8 hours.
3. Add bell pepper, onions, and oil to the marinade and mix well.
4. Yarn the chicken, peppers, and onions on the skewers.
5. Set the air fryer basket.
6. Hit the "Air Fryer Button" and select 10 minutes of cooking time, then press "Start."
7. Once the air fryer oven beeps, flip the skewers and continue air frying for 7 minutes.
8. Serve.

Nutrition:

- Calories: 241
- Total Fat: 14.2 g
- Saturated Fat: 3.8 g
- Cholesterol: 92 mg
- Sodium: 695 mg
- Total Carbs: 8.5 g
- Dietary Fiber: 1.6 g
- Total Sugars: 3.9 g
- Protein: 21.8 g

23. CREAMY CHICKEN THIGHS

Preparation Time: 10 minutes

Cooking Time: 30 minutes

Servings: 2

Ingredients:

- » 1 tbsp. olive oil
- » 6 chicken thighs, bone-in, skin-on
- » Salt
- » Freshly ground black pepper
- » 3/4 cup low-sodium chicken broth
- » 1/2 cup heavy cream
- » 1/2 cup sun-dried tomatoes, chopped
- » 1/4 cup Parmesan, grated
- » Freshly torn basil to serve

Directions:

1. Stir in chicken, salt, and black pepper, then sear for 5 minutes per side.
2. Add broth, cream, parmesan, and tomatoes.
3. Select 20 minutes of cooking time, then press "Start."
4. Once the Air Fryer oven beeps, garnish with basil and serve.
5. Enjoy

Nutrition:

- Calories 454
- Total Fat 37.8g
- Saturated Fat 14.4g
- Cholesterol 169mg
- Sodium: 181 mg
- Total Carbs: 2.8 g
- Dietary Fiber: 0.7 g
- Total Sugars: 0.7 g
- Protein: 26.9 g

Chapter 6.

BEEF RECIPES

24. MEATLOAF SLIDER WRAPS

Preparation Time: 15 minutes

Cooking Time: 10 minutes

Servings: 2

Ingredients:

» 1 pound ground beef, grass-fed
» 1/2 cup almond flour
» 1/4 cup coconut flour
» 1/2 tbsp. minced garlic
» 1/4 cup chopped white onion
» 1 tsp. Italian seasoning
» 1/2 tsp. sea salt
» 1/2 tsp. dried tarragon
» 1/2 tsp. ground black pepper
» 1 tbsp. Worcestershire sauce
» 1/4 cup ketchup
» 2 eggs, pastured, beaten
» 1 head of lettuce

Directions:

1. Place all the ingredients in a bowl, stir well, then shape the mixture into 2-inch diameters and 1-inch thick patties and refrigerate them for 10 minutes.
2. Meanwhile, switch on the air fryer, insert the fryer basket, grease it with olive oil, then shut with its lid, set the fryer at 360°F, and preheat for 10 minutes.
3. Open the fryer, add patties to it in a single layer, close with its lid and cook for 10 minutes until nicely golden and cooked, flipping the patties halfway through the frying.
4. When the air fryer beeps, open its lid and transfer patties to a plate.
5. Wrap each patty in lettuce and serve.

Nutrition:

- Calories: 228
- Carbs: 6 g
- Fat: 16 g
- Protein: 13 g
- Fiber: 2 g

25. DOUBLE CHEESEBURGER

Preparation Time: 5 minutes

Cooking Time: 18 minutes

Servings: 1

Ingredients:

» 2 beef patties, pastured
» 1/8 tsp. onion powder
» 2 slices of mozzarella cheese, low-fat
» 1/8 tsp. ground black pepper
» 1/8 tsp. salt
» 2 tbsp of olive oil

Directions:

1. Switch on the air fryer, insert the basket, grease it with olive oil, set the fryer at 370°F and, preheat for 5 minutes.
2. Meanwhile, season the patties well with onion powder, black pepper, and salt.
3. Open the fryer, add beef patties in it, close with its lid and cook for 12 minutes until nicely golden and cooked, flipping the patties halfway through the frying.
4. Then top the patties with a cheese slice and continue cooking for 1 minute or until cheese melts.
5. Serve straight away.

Nutrition:

- Calories: 670
- Carbs: 0 g
- Fat: 50 g
- Protein: 39 g
- Fiber: 0 g

26. BEEF SCHNITZEL

Preparation Time: 10 minutes

Cooking Time: 15 minutes

Servings: 1

Ingredients:

» 1 lean beef schnitzel
» 2 tbsp. olive oil
» 1/4 cup breadcrumbs
» 1 egg
» 1 lemon and salad greens to serve

Directions:

1. Let the air fryer heat to 180°C.
2. In a big bowl, add breadcrumbs and oil, mix well until it forms a crumbly mixture.
3. Dip beef steak in whisked egg and coat in breadcrumbs mixture.
4. Place the breaded beef in the air fryer and cook at 180C for 15 minutes or more until fully cooked through.
5. Take out from the air fryer and serve with the side of salad greens and lemon.

Nutrition:

- Calories: 340
- Proteins: 20 g
- Carbs: 14 g
- Fat: 10 g
- Fiber: 7 g

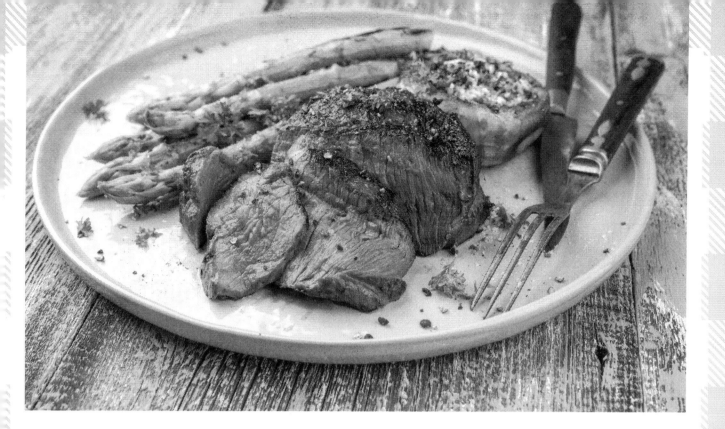

27. STEAK WITH ASPARAGUS BUNDLES

Preparation Time: 20 minutes

Cooking Time: 30 minutes

Servings: 2

Ingredients:

» Olive oil spray
» 2 lb. flank steak, cut into 6 pieces
» Kosher salt and black pepper
» 2 cloves minced garlic
» 4 cups asparagus
» 1/2 Tamari sauce
» 3 bell peppers sliced thinly
» 1/3 cup beef broth
» 1 tbsp. unsalted butter
» 1/4 cup balsamic vinegar

Directions:

1. Sprinkle salt and pepper on steak and rub.
2. In a Ziploc bag, add garlic and Tamari sauce, then add steak, toss well and seal the bag.
3. Let it marinate for 1 hour or overnight.
4. Equally, place bell peppers and asparagus in the center of the steak.
5. Roll the steak around the vegetables and secure well with toothpicks.
6. Preheat the air fryer.
7. Drizzle the steak with olive oil spray. And place steaks in the air fryer.
8. Cook for 15 minutes at 400°F or more until steaks are cooked.
9. Take the steak out from the air fryer and let it rest for 5 minutes.
10. Remove steak bundles and allow them to rest for 5 minutes before serving and slicing.
11. In the meantime, add butter, balsamic vinegar, and broth over medium flame. Mix well and reduce it by half. Add salt and pepper to taste.
12. Pour over steaks right before serving.

Nutrition:

- Calories: 471
- Proteins: 29 g
- Carbs: 20 g
- Fat: 15 g

28. HAMBURGERS

Preparation Time: 5 minutes

Cooking Time: 6 minutes

Servings: 4

Ingredients:

- » 4 buns
- » 4 cups lean ground beef chuck
- » Salt to taste
- » 4 slices any cheese
- » Black Pepper to taste
- » 2 sliced tomatoes
- » 1 head of lettuce
- » Ketchup for dressing

Directions:

1. Let the air fryer preheat to 350°F.
2. In a bowl, add lean ground beef, pepper, and salt. Mix well and form patties.
3. Put them in the air fryer in one layer only, cook for 6 minutes, flip them halfway through. 1 minute before you take out the patties, add cheese on top.
4. When cheese is melted, take it out from the air fryer.
5. Add ketchup or any dressing to your buns; add tomatoes, lettuce, and patties.
6. Serve hot.

Nutrition:

- Calories: 520
- Carbs: 22 g
- Protein: 31 g
- Fat: 34 g

29. BEEF STEAK KABOBS WITH VEGETABLES

Preparation Time: 30 minutes

Cooking Time: 10 minutes

Servings: 4

Ingredients:

- » 2 tbsp. light soy sauce
- » 4 cups lean beef chuck ribs, cut into 1-inch pieces
- » 1/3 cup low-fat sour cream
- » 1/2 onion
- » 8 6-inch skewers
- » 1 bell pepper
- » Black pepper
- » Yogurt for dipping

Directions:

1. In a mixing bowl, add soy sauce and sour cream, mix well. Add the lean beef chunks, coat well, and let it marinate for half an hour or more.
2. Cut onion, bell pepper into 1-inch pieces. In water, soak skewers for 10 minutes.
3. Add onions, bell peppers, and beef on skewers; alternatively, sprinkle with black pepper.
4. Let it cook for 10 minutes in a preheated air fryer at 400°F, flip halfway through.
5. Serve with yogurt dipping sauce.

Nutrition:

- Calories: 268
- Proteins: 20 g
- Carbs: 15 g
- Fat: 10 g

30. RIB-EYE STEAK

Preparation Time: 5 minutes

Cooking Time: 14 minutes

Servings: 2

Ingredients:

» 2 lean ribeye steaks medium-sized
» Salt and freshly ground black pepper to taste
» Microgreen salad to serve

Directions:

1. Let the air fryer preheat at 400°F. Pat dry steaks with paper towels.
2. Use any spice blend or just salt and pepper on steaks.
3. Generously on both sides of the steak.
4. Put steaks in the air fryer basket. Cook according to the rareness you want. Or cook for 14 minutes and flip after halftime.
5. Take out from the air fryer and let it rest for about 5 minutes.
6. Serve with microgreen salad.

Nutrition:

- Calories: 470
- Protein: 45 g
- Fat: 31 g
- Carbs: 23 g

31. BUNLESS SLOPPY JOES

Preparation Time: 15 minutes

Cooking Time: 40 minutes

Servings: 2

Ingredients:

» 6 small sweet potatoes
» 1 pound (454 g) lean ground beef
» 1 onion, finely chopped
» 1 carrot, finely chopped
» 1/4 cup finely chopped mushrooms
» 1/4 cup finely chopped red bell pepper
» 3 garlic cloves, minced
» 2 tsp. Worcestershire sauce
» 1 tbsp. white wine vinegar
» 1 (15 oz./425 g) can low-sodium tomato sauce
» 2 tbsp. tomato paste

Directions:

1. Preheat the air fryer oven to 400°F (205°C).
2. Place the sweet potatoes in a single layer in a baking dish. Bake for 25 to 40 minutes, depending on the size, until they are soft and cooked through.
3. While the sweet potatoes are baking in a large skillet, cook the beef over medium heat until it's browned, breaking it apart into small pieces as you stir.
4. Add the onion, carrot, mushrooms, bell pepper, and garlic, and saute briefly for 1 minute.
5. Stir in the Worcestershire sauce, vinegar, tomato sauce, and tomato paste. Bring to a simmer, reduce the heat, and cook for 5 minutes for the flavors to meld.
6. Scoop ½ cup of the meat mixture on top of each baked potato and serve.

Nutrition:

- Calories: 372
- Fat: 19 g
- Protein: 16 g
- Carbs: 34 g
- Sugars: 13 g
- Fiber: 6 g
- Sodium: 161 mg

32. BEEF CURRY

Preparation Time: 15 minutes

Cooking Time: 10 minutes

Servings: 2

Ingredients:

» 1 tbsp. extra-virgin olive oil
» 1 small onion, thinly sliced
» 2 tsp. minced fresh ginger
» 3 garlic cloves, minced
» 2 tsp. ground coriander
» 1 tsp. ground cumin
» 1 jalapeño or serrano pepper, split lengthwise but not all the way through
» 1/4 tsp. ground turmeric
» 1/4 tsp. salt
» 1 lb. (454 g) grass-fed sirloin tip steak, top round steak, or top sirloin steak, cut into bite-size pieces
» 2 tbsp. chopped fresh cilantro
» 1/4 cup water

Directions:

1. In an air fryer oven, heat the oil over medium-high.
2. Add the onion, and cook for 3 to 5 minutes until browned and softened. Add the ginger and garlic, stirring continuously until fragrant, about 30 seconds.
3. In a small bowl, mix the coriander, cumin, jalapeño, turmeric, and salt. Add the spice mixture to the skillet and stir continuously for 1 minute. Deglaze the skillet with about ¼ cup of water.
4. Add the beef and stir continuously for about 5 minutes until well-browned yet still medium-rare. Remove the jalapeño. Serve topped with cilantro.

Nutrition:

- Calories: 140
- Fat: 7 g
- Protein: 18 g
- Carbs: 3 g
- Sugars: 1 g
- Fiber: 1 g
- Sodium: 141 mg

33. BEEF BURRITO BOWL

Preparation Time: 5 minutes

Cooking Time: 10 minutes

Servings: 4

Ingredients:

» 1 lb. (454 g) 93% lean ground beef
» 1 cup canned low-sodium black beans, drained and rinsed
» 1/4 tsp. ground cumin
» 1/4 tsp. chili powder
» 1/4 tsp. garlic powder
» 1/4 tsp. onion powder
» 1/4 tsp. salt
» 1 head romaine or preferred lettuce, shredded
» 2 medium tomatoes, chopped
» 1 cup shredded Cheddar cheese or packaged cheese blend

Directions:

1. Preheat the air fryer oven to 400°F (205°C).
2. Put the beef, beans, cumin, chili powder, garlic powder, onion powder, and salt into the skillet, and cook for 8 to 10 minutes until cooked through. Stir occasionally.
3. Divide the lettuce evenly between four bowls. Add 1/4 of the beef mixture to each bowl and top with 1/4 of the tomatoes and cheese.

Nutrition:

- Calories: 351
- Fat: 18 g
- Protein: 35 g
- Carbs: 14 g
- Sugars: 4 g
- Fiber: 6 g
- Sodium: 424 mg

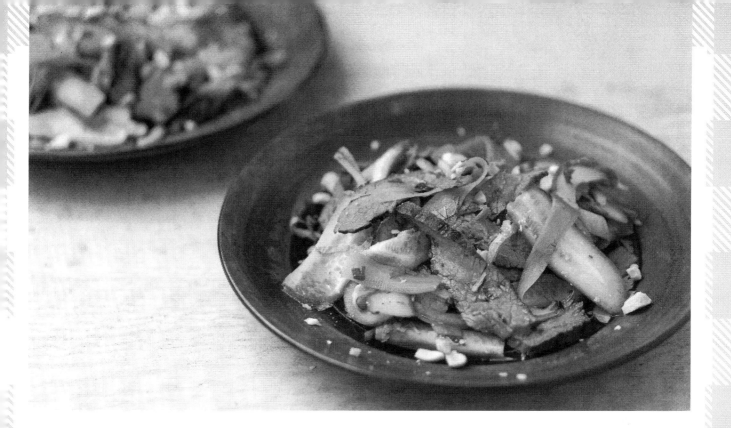

34. ASIAN GRILLED BEEF SALAD

Preparation Time: 15 minutes

Cooking Time: 15 minutes

Servings: 4

Ingredients:

Dressing:
- » 1/4 cup freshly squeezed lime juice
- » 1 tbsp. low-sodium tamari or gluten-free soy sauce
- » 1 tbsp. extra-virgin olive oil
- » 1 garlic clove, minced
- » 1 tsp. honey
- » 1/4 tsp. red pepper flakes

Salad:
- » 1 lb. (454 g) grass-fed flank steak
- » 1/4 tsp. salt
- » Pinch freshly ground black pepper
- » 6 cups chopped leaf lettuce
- » 1 cucumber, halved lengthwise and thinly cut into half-moons
- » 1/2 small red onion, sliced
- » 1 carrot, cut into ribbons
- » 1/4 cup chopped fresh cilantro

Directions:

Make the Dressing:
1. In a small bowl, whisk together the lime juice, tamari, olive oil, garlic, honey, and red pepper flakes. Set aside.

Make the Salad:
2. Season the beef on both sides with salt and pepper.
3. Preheat the air fryer oven to 400°F (205°C).
4. Cook the beef for 3 to 6 minutes per side, depending on preferred doneness. Set aside, tented with aluminum foil, for 10 minutes.
5. In a large bowl, toss the lettuce, cucumber, onion, carrot, and cilantro.
6. Slice the beef thinly against the grain and transfer to the salad bowl.
7. Drizzle with the dressing and toss. Serve.

Nutrition:

- Calories: 231
- Fat: 10 g
- Protein: 26 g
- Carbs: 10 g
- Sugars: 4 g
- Fiber: 2 g
- Sodium: 349 mg

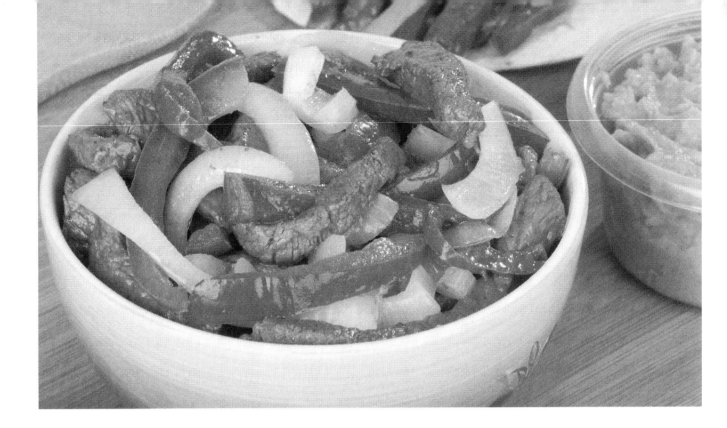

35. BEEF AND PEPPER FAJITA BOWLS

Preparation Time: 10 minutes

Cooking Time: 15 minutes

Servings: 4

Ingredients:

- » 4 tbsp. extra-virgin olive oil, divided
- » 1 head cauliflower, riced
- » 1 lb. (454 g) sirloin steak, cut into ¼-inch-thick strips
- » 1 red bell pepper, seeded and sliced
- » 1 onion, thinly sliced
- » 2 garlic cloves, minced
- » 2 limes juice
- » 1 tsp. chili powder

Directions:

1. Preheat the air fryer oven to 400°F (205°C).
2. Heat 2 tablespoons of olive oil until it shimmers.
3. Add the cauliflower. Cook, stirring occasionally, until it softens, about 3 minutes. Set aside.
4. Add the remaining 2 tablespoons of oil to the air fryer, and heat it on medium-high until it shimmers.
5. Add the steak and cook, stirring occasionally, until it browns, about 3 minutes. Use a slotted spoon to remove the steak from the oil in the pan and set it aside.
6. Add the bell pepper and onion to the pan. Cook, stirring occasionally, until they start to brown, about 5 minutes.
7. Add the garlic and cook, stirring constantly, for 30 seconds.
8. Return the beef along with any juices that have been collected and the cauliflower to the pan. Add the lime juice and chili powder. Cook, stirring, until everything is warmed through, 2 to 3 minutes.

Nutrition:

- Calories: 310
- Fat: 18 g
- Protein: 27 g
- Carbs: 13 g
- Sugars: 2 g
- Fiber: 3 g
- Sodium: 93 mg

Chapter 7.

PORK RECIPES

36. COUNTRY-STYLE PORK RIBS

Preparation Time: 5 minutes

Cooking Time: 20–25 minutes

Servings: 4

Ingredients:

- » 12 country-style pork ribs, trimmed excess fat
- » 2 tbsp. cornstarch
- » 2 tbsp. olive oil
- » 1 tsp. dry mustard
- » 1/2 tsp. thyme
- » 1/2 tsp. garlic powder
- » 1 tsp. dried marjoram
- » Pinch salt
- » Freshly ground black pepper, to taste

Directions:

1. Place the ribs on a clean work surface.
2. In a small bowl, combine the cornstarch, olive oil, mustard, thyme, garlic powder, marjoram, salt, and pepper, and rub into the ribs.
3. Place the ribs in the air fryer basket and roast at 400°F (204°C) for 10 minutes.
4. Carefully, turn the ribs using tongs and roast for 10 to 15 minutes or until the ribs are crisp and register an internal temperature of at least 150°F (66°C).

Nutrition:

- Calories: 579
- Fat: 44 g
- Protein: 40 g
- Carbs: 4 g
- Fiber: 0 g
- Sugar: 0 g
- Sodium: 155 mg

37. LEMON AND HONEY PORK TENDERLOIN

Preparation Time: 5 minutes

Cooking Time: 10 minutes

Servings: 4

Ingredients:

» 1 (1 pound/454 g) pork tenderloin, cut into ½-inch slices
» 1 tbsp. olive oil
» 1 tbsp. freshly squeezed lemon juice
» 1 tbsp. honey
» 1/2 tsp. grated lemon zest
» 1/2 tsp. dried marjoram
» Pinch salt
» Freshly ground black pepper to taste

Directions:

1. Put the pork tenderloin slices in a medium bowl.
2. In a small bowl, combine the olive oil, lemon juice, honey, lemon zest, marjoram, salt, and pepper. Mix.
3. Pour this marinade over the tenderloin slices and massage gently with your hands to work it into the pork.
4. Place the pork in the air fryer basket and roast at 400°F (204°C) for 10 minutes or until the pork registers at least 145°F (63°C) using a meat thermometer.

Nutrition:

- Calories: 208
- Fat: 8 g
- Protein: 30 g
- Carbs: 5 g
- Fiber: 0 g
- Sugar: 4 g
- Sodium: 104 mg

38. DIJON PORK TENDERLOIN

Preparation Time: 10 minutes

Cooking Time: 12–14 minutes

Servings: 4

Ingredients:

» 1 lb. (454 g) pork tenderloin, cut into 1-inch slices
» Pinch salt
» Freshly ground black pepper to taste
» 2 tbsp. Dijon mustard
» 1 garlic clove, minced
» 1/2 tsp. dried basil
» 1 cup soft bread crumbs
» 2 tbsp. olive oil

Directions:

1. Slightly pound the pork slices until they are about ¾ inch thick. Sprinkle with salt and pepper on both sides.
2. Coat the pork with the Dijon mustard and sprinkle with garlic and basil.
3. On a plate, combine the bread crumbs and olive oil and mix well. Coat the pork slices with the bread crumb mixture, patting, so the crumbs adhere.
4. Place the pork in the air fryer basket, leaving a little space between each piece. Air fry at 390°F (199°C) for 12 to 14 minutes or until the pork reaches at least 145°F (63°C) on a meat thermometer, and the coating is crisp and brown. Serve immediately.

Nutrition:

- Calories: 336
- Fat: 13 g
- Protein: 34 g
- Carbs: 20 g
- Fiber: 2 g
- Sugar: 2 g
- Sodium: 390 mg

39. PORK SATAY

Preparation Time: 15 minutes

Cooking Time: 9–14 minutes

Servings: 4

Ingredients:

» 1 (1 lb. / 454 g) pork tenderloin, cut into 1½-inch cubes
» 1/4 cup minced onion
» 2 garlic cloves, minced
» 1 jalapeño pepper, minced
» 2 tbsp. freshly squeezed lime juice
» 2 tbsp. coconut milk
» 2 tbsp. unsalted peanut butter
» 2 tsp. curry powder

Directions:

1. In a medium bowl, mix the pork, onion, garlic, jalapeño, lime juice, coconut milk, peanut butter, and curry powder until well combined. Let stand for 10 minutes at room temperature.
2. With a slotted spoon, remove the pork from the marinade. Reserve the marinade.
3. Thread the pork onto about 8 bamboo or metal skewers. Air fry at 380°F (193°C) for 9 to 14 minutes, brushing once with the reserved marinade until the pork reaches at least 145°F (63°C) on a meat thermometer. Discard any remaining marinade. Serve immediately.

Nutrition:

- Calories: 195
- Fat: 7 g
- Protein: 25 g
- Carbs: 7 g
- Fiber: 1 g
- Sugar: 3 g
- Sodium: 65 mg

40. PORK BURGERS WITH RED CABBAGE SLAW

Preparation Time: 20 minutes

Cooking Time: 7–9 minutes

Servings: 4

Ingredients:

» 1/2 cup Greek yogurt
» 2 tbsp. low-sodium mustard, divided
» 1 tbsp. freshly squeezed lemon juice
» 1/4 cup sliced red cabbage
» 1/4 cup grated carrots
» 1 pound (454 g) lean ground pork
» 1/2 tsp. paprika
» 1 cup mixed baby lettuce greens
» 2 small tomatoes, sliced
» 8 small low-sodium whole-wheat sandwich buns, cut in half

Directions:

1. In a small bowl, combine the yogurt, 1 tablespoon mustard, lemon juice, cabbage, and carrots; mix and refrigerate.
2. In a medium bowl, combine the pork, the remaining 1 tablespoon mustard, and paprika. Form into 8 small patties.
3. Put the patties into the air fryer basket. Air fry at 400°F (204°C) for 7 to 9 minutes, or until the patties register 165°F (74°C) as tested with a meat thermometer.
4. Assemble the burgers by placing some of the lettuce greens on a bun bottom. Top with a tomato slice, the patties, and the cabbage mixture. Add the bun top and serve immediately.

Nutrition:

- Calories: 473
- Fat: 15 g
- Protein: 35 g
- Carbs: 51 g
- Fiber: 8 g
- Sugar: 8 g
- Sodium: 138 mg

41. BREADED PORK CHOPS

Preparation Time: 10 minutes

Cooking Time: 12 minutes

Servings: 4

Ingredients:

» 1 cup Whole-wheat breadcrumbs
» Salt ¼ tsp.
» 2–4 pcs. pork chops (center cut and boneless)
» 1/2 tsp. chili powder
» 1 tbsp. parmesan cheese
» 1½ tsp. paprika
» 1 egg beaten
» 1/2 tsp. onion powder
» 1/2 tsp. grounded garlic
» Pepper to taste

Directions:

1. Let the air fryer preheat to 400°F
2. Rub kosher salt on each side of pork chops, let it rest
3. Add beaten egg in a big bowl
4. Add Parmesan cheese, breadcrumbs, garlic, pepper, paprika, chili powder, and onion powder in a bowl and mix well
5. Dip pork chop in egg, then in breadcrumb mixture
6. Put it in the air fryer and spray it with oil.
7. Let it cook for 12 minutes at 400°F. Flip it over halfway through. Cook for another 6 minutes.
8. Serve with a side of salad.

Nutrition:

- Calories: 425
- Fat: 20 g
- Fiber: 5 g
- Protein: 31 g
- Carbs: 19 g

42. PORK TAQUITOS IN AIR FRYER

Preparation Time: 10 minutes

Cooking Time: 7-10 minutes

Servings: 2

Ingredients:

» 3 cups pork tenderloin, cooked and shredded
» Cooking spray
» 2 ½ shredded mozzarella, fat-free
» 10 small tortillas
» 1 lime juice

Directions:

1. Let the air fryer preheat to 380°F.
2. Add lime juice to pork and mix well.
3. With a damp towel over the tortilla, microwave for 10 seconds to soften.
4. Add pork filling and cheese on top in a tortilla, roll up the tortilla tightly.
5. Place tortillas on a greased foil pan
6. Spray oil over tortillas. Cook for 7 to 10 minutes or until tortillas are golden brown, flip halfway through.
7. Serve with fresh salad.

Nutrition:

- Calories: 253
- Fat: 18 g
- Carbs: 10 g
- Protein: 20 g

43. TASTY EGG ROLLS

Preparation Time: 10 minutes

Cooking Time: 20 minutes

Servings: 3

Ingredients:

- » 1/2 bag coleslaw mix
- » 1/2 onion
- » 1/2 tsp. salt
- » 1/2 cup mushrooms
- » Lean ground pork: 2 cups
- » 1 stalk celery
- » 12 Wrappers (egg roll)

Directions:

1. Put a skillet over medium flame, add onion and lean ground pork and cook for 5 to 7 minutes.
2. Add coleslaw mixture, salt, mushrooms, and celery to skillet and cook for almost 5 minutes.
3. Lay egg roll wrapper flat and add filling (1/3 cup), roll it up, seal with water.
4. Spray with oil the rolls.
5. Put in the air fryer for 6 to 8 minutes at 400°F, flipping once halfway through.
6. Serve hot.

Nutrition:

- Calories: 245
- Fat: 10 g
- Carbs: 9 g
- Protein: 11 g

44. PORK DUMPLINGS

Preparation Time: 30 minutes

Cooking Time: 20 minutes

Servings: 4

Ingredients:

- » 18 dumpling wrappers
- » 1 tsp. olive oil
- » 4 cups bok choy (chopped)
- » 2 tbsp. rice vinegar
- » 1 tbsp. diced ginger
- » 1/4 tsp. crushed red pepper
- » 1 tbsp. diced garlic
- » 1/2 cup lean ground pork
- » Cooking spray
- » 2 tsp. lite soy sauce
- » 1/2 tsp. honey
- » 1 tsp. Toasted sesame oil
- » 1/8 cup finely chopped scallions

Directions:

1. Preheat the air fryer oven to 400°F (205°C).
2. Add bok choy, cook for 6 minutes, and add garlic, ginger, and cook for 1 minute. Move this mixture on a paper towel, and pat dry the excess oil
3. In a bowl, add bok choy mixture, crushed pepper, and lean ground pork and mix well.
4. Lay a dumpling wrapper on a plate and add 1 tablespoon of filling in the wrapper's middle. With water, seal the edges and crimp them.
5. Spray oil on the air fryer basket, add dumplings in it and cook at 375°F for 12 minutes or until browned.
6. In the meantime, to make the sauce, add sesame oil, rice vinegar, scallions, soy sauce, and honey in a bowl mix together.
7. Serve the dumplings with sauce.

Nutrition:

- Calories: 140
- Fat: 5 g
- Protein: 12 g
- Carbs: 9 g

45. PORK CHOP & BROCCOLI

Preparation Time: 20 minutes

Cooking Time: 10 minutes

Servings: 2

Ingredients:

- » 2 cups broccoli florets
- » 2 pcs. bone-in pork chop
- » 1/2 tsp. paprika
- » 2 tbsp. avocado oil
- » 1/2 tsp. garlic powder
- » 1/2 tsp. onion powder
- » 2 cloves crushed garlic
- » 1 tsp. salt divided
- » Cooking spray

Directions:

1. Let the air fryer preheat to 350°F. Spray the basket with cooking oil
2. Add 1 tablespoon avocado oil, onion powder, ½ teaspoon of salt, garlic powder, and paprika in a bowl, mix well, rub this spice mix to the pork chop's sides
3. Add pork chops to air fryer basket and let it cook for 5 minutes
4. In the meantime, add 1 remaining teaspoon of avocado oil, garlic, the other ½ teaspoon of salt, and broccoli to a bowl and coat well
5. Flip the pork chop and add the broccoli. Let it cook for 5 more minutes.
6. Take out from the air fryer and serve.

Nutrition:

- Calories: 483
- Fat: 20 g
- Carbs: 12 g
- Protein: 23 g

46. CHEESY PORK CHOPS

Preparation Time: 5 minutes

Cooking Time: 4 minutes

Servings: 2

Ingredients:

- » 4 lean pork chops
- » 1/2 tsp. salt
- » 1/2 tsp. garlic powder
- » 4 tbsp. shredded cheese
- » 2 chopped cilantros

Directions:

1. Let the air fryer preheat to 350°F.
2. With garlic, cilantro, and salt, rub the pork chops. Put in the air fryer. Let it cook for 4 minutes.
3. Flip them and cook for 2 more minutes.
4. Add cheese on top of them and cook for another 2 minutes or until the cheese is melted.
5. Serve with salad greens.

Nutrition:

- Calories: 467
- Protein: 61 g
- Fat: 22 g
- Saturated Fat: 8 g

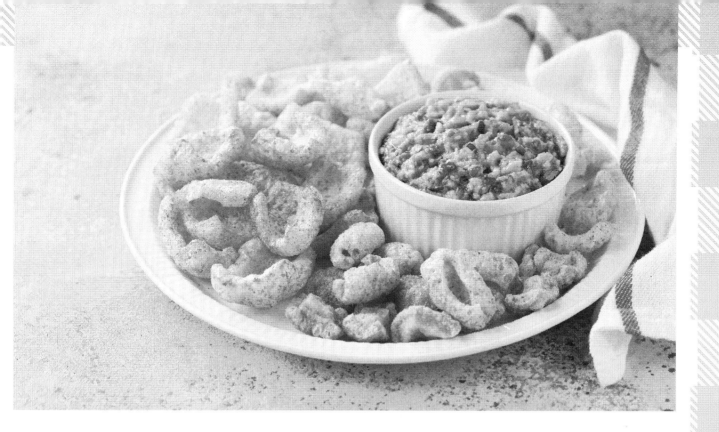

47. PORK RIND NACHOS

Preparation Time: 5 minutes

Cooking Time: 5 minutes

Servings: 2

Ingredients:

- » 2 tbsp. pork rinds
- » 1/4 cup shredded cooked chicken
- » 1/2 cup shredded Monterey jack cheese
- » 1/4 cup sliced pickled jalapeños
- » 1/4 cup guacamole
- » 1/4 cup full-fat sour cream

Nutrition:

- Calories: 295
- Protein: 30.1 g
- Fiber: 1.2 g
- Carbs: 1.8 g
- Fat: 27.5 g
- Carbs: 3.0 g

Directions:

1. Put pork rinds in a 6-inches round baking pan. Fill with grilled chicken and Monterey cheese jack. Place the pan in the basket with the air fryer.
2. Set the temperature to 370°F and set the timer for 5 minutes or until the cheese has been melted.
3. Eat right away with jalapeños, guacamole, and sour cream.

Chapter 8.

LAMB RECIPES

48. GREEK LAMB PITA POCKETS

Preparation Time: 15 minutes

Cooking Time: 5–7 minutes

Servings: 4

Ingredients:

Dressing:
» 1 cup plain Greek yogurt
» 1 tbsp. lemon juice
» 1 tsp. dried dill weed, crushed
» 1 tsp. ground oregano
» 1/2 tsp. salt

Meatballs:
» 1/2-pound (227 g) ground lamb
» 1 tbsp. diced onion
» 1 tsp. dried parsley
» 1 tsp. dried dill weed, crushed
» 1/4 tsp. oregano
» 1/4 tsp. coriander
» 1/4 tsp. ground cumin
» 1/4 tsp. salt
» 4 pita halves

Suggested Toppings:
» Red onion, slivered
» Seedless cucumber, thinly sliced
» Crumbled feta cheese
» Sliced black olives
» Chopped fresh peppers

Directions:

1. Stir dressing ingredients together and refrigerate while preparing lamb.
2. Combine all meatball ingredients in a large bowl and stir to distribute seasonings.
3. Shape meat mixture into 12 small meatballs, rounded or slightly flattened if you prefer.
4. Air fry at 390°F (199°C) for 5 to 7 minutes, until well done. Remove and drain on paper towels.
5. To serve, pile meatballs and your choice of toppings in pita pockets and drizzle with dressing.

Nutrition:
- Calories: 270
- Fat: 14 g
- Protein: 18 g
- Carbs: 18 g
- Fiber: 2 g
- Sugar: 2 g
- Sodium: 618 mg

49. ROSEMARY LAMB CHOPS

Preparation Time: 30 minutes

Cooking Time: 20 minutes

Servings: 2-3

Ingredients:

- » 2 tsp. oil
- » 1/2 tsp. ground rosemary
- » 1/2 tsp. lemon juice
- » 1 lb. (454 g) lamb chops, approximately 1-inch thick
- » Salt and pepper to taste
- » Cooking spray

Directions:

1. Mix the oil, rosemary, and lemon juice and rub into all sides of the lamb chops. Season to taste with salt and pepper.
2. For best flavor, cover lamb chops and allow them to rest in the fridge for 15 to 20 minutes.
3. Spray air fryer basket with non-stick spray and place lamb chops in it.
4. Air fry at 360°F (182°C) for approximately 20 minutes. This will cook chops to medium. The meat will be juicy but have no remaining pink. Air fry for 1 to 2 minutes longer for well-done chops. For rare chops, continue cooking for about 12 minutes and check for doneness.

Nutrition:

- Calories: 237
- Fat: 13 g
- Protein: 30 g
- Carbs: 0 g
- Fiber: 0 g
- Sugar 0 g
- Sodium: 116 mg

50. HERB BUTTER LAMB CHOPS

Preparation Time: 10 minutes

Cooking Time: 5 minutes

Servings: 4

Ingredients:

- » 4 lamb chops
- » 1 tsp. rosemary, diced
- » 1 tbsp. butter
- » Pepper
- » Salt

Directions:

1. Season lamb chops with pepper and salt.
2. Place the dehydrating tray in a multi-level air fryer basket and insert the basket in the air fryer oven.
3. Place lamb chops on dehydrating tray.
4. Seal pot with air fryer lid and select "Air Fry" mode, then set the temperature to 400°F and timer for 5 minutes.
5. Mix butter and rosemary and spread overcooked lamb chops.
6. Serve and enjoy.

Nutrition:

- Calories: 278
- Cholesterol: 129 mg
- Fat: 12.8 g
- Carbs: 0.2 g
- Sugar: 0 g
- Protein: 38 g

51. ZA'ATAR LAMB CHOPS

Preparation Time: 10 minutes

Cooking Time: 10 minutes

Servings: 4

Ingredients:

- » 4 lamb loin chops
- » 1/2 tbsp. Za'atar
- » 1 tbsp. fresh lemon juice
- » 1 tsp. olive oil
- » 2 garlic cloves, minced
- » Pepper
- » Salt

Directions:

1. Coat lamb chops with oil and lemon juice and rubs with Za'atar, garlic, pepper, and salt.
2. Place the dehydrating tray in a multi-level air fryer basket and insert the basket in the air fryer oven.
3. Place lamb chops on dehydrating tray.
4. Seal pot with air fryer lid and select air fry mode, then set the temperature to 400°F and timer for 10 minutes. Turn lamb chops halfway through.
5. Serve and enjoy.

Nutrition:

- Calories: 266
- Fat: 11.2 g
- Carbs: 0.6 g
- Cholesterol: 122 mg
- Sugar: 0.1 g
- Protein: 38 g

52. GREEK LAMB CHOPS

Preparation Time: 10 minutes

Cooking Time: 10 minutes

Servings: 4

Ingredients:

- » 2 lb. lamb chops
- » 2 tsp. garlic, minced
- » 1 ½ tsp. dried oregano
- » 1/4 cup fresh lemon juice
- » 1/4 cup olive oil
- » 1/2 tsp. pepper
- » 1 tsp. salt

Directions:

1. Add lamb chops in a mixing bowl. Add remaining ingredients over the lamb chops and coat well.
2. Arrange lamb chops on the air fryer oven tray and cook at 400°F for 5 minutes.
3. Turn lamb chops and cook for 5 more minutes.
4. Serve and enjoy.

Nutrition:

- Calories: 538
- Fat: 29.4 g
- Carbs: 1.3 g
- Protein: 64 g

53.   HERBED LAMB CHOPS

Preparation Time: 1 hour 10 minutes

Cooking Time: 13 minutes

Servings: 4

Ingredients:

- »   1 lb. lamb chops, pastured
- »   For the Marinate:
- »   2 tbsp. lemon juice
- »   1 tsp. dried rosemary
- »   1 tsp. salt
- »   1 tsp. dried thyme
- »   1 tsp. coriander
- »   1 tsp. dried oregano
- »   2 tbsp. olive oil

Directions:

1. Prepare the marinade and for this, place all its ingredients in a bowl and whisk until combined.
2. Pour the marinade into a large plastic bag, add lamb chops in it, seal the bag, then turn it upside down to coat lamb chops with the marinade and let it in the refrigerator for a minimum of 1 hour.
3. Then switch on the air fryer, insert fryer basket, grease it with olive oil, then shut with its lid, set the fryer at 390°F, and preheat for 5 minutes.
4. Open the fryer, add marinated lamb chops in it, close with its lid and cook for 8 minutes until nicely golden and cooked, turning the lamb chops halfway through the frying.
5. When the air fryer beeps, open its lid, transfer lamb chops to a plate and serve.

Nutrition:

- Calories: 177.4
- Carbs: 1.7 g
- Fat: 8 g
- Protein: 23.4 g
- Fiber: 0.5 g

54.   SPICY LAMB SIRLOIN STEAK

Preparation Time: 40 minutes

Cooking Time: 20 minutes

Servings: 4

Ingredients:

- »   1 lb. lamb sirloin steaks, pastured, boneless
- »   For the Marinade:
- »   1/2 white onion, peeled
- »   1 tsp. ground fennel
- »   5 garlic cloves, peeled
- »   4 slices ginger
- »   1 tsp. salt
- »   1/2 tsp. ground cardamom
- »   1 tsp. garam masala
- »   1 tsp. ground cinnamon
- »   1 tsp. cayenne pepper

Directions:

1. Place all the ingredients for the marinade in a food processor and then pulse until well blended.
2. Make cuts in the lamb chops by using a knife, then place them in a large bowl and add prepared marinade in it.
3. Mix well until lamb chops are coated with the marinade and let them in the refrigerator for a minimum of 30 minutes.
4. Then switch on the air fryer, insert fryer basket, grease it with olive oil, then shut with its lid, set the fryer at 330°F, and preheat for 5 minutes.
5. Open the fryer, add lamb chops in it, close with its lid and cook for 15 minutes until nicely golden and cooked, flipping the steaks halfway through the frying.
6. When the air fryer beeps, open its lid, transfer lamb steaks to a plate and serve.

Nutrition:

- Calories: 182
- Carbs: 3 g
- Fat: 7 g
- Protein: 24 g
- Fiber: 1 g

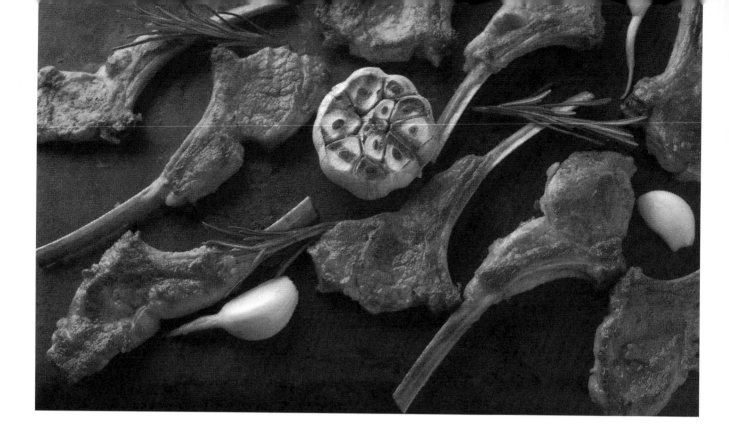

55. GARLIC ROSEMARY LAMB CHOPS

Preparation Time: 1 hour 10 minutes

Cooking Time: 12 minutes

Servings: 4

Ingredients:

» 4 lamb chops, pastured
» 1 tsp. ground black pepper
» 2 tsp. minced garlic
» 1 ½ tsp. salt
» 2 tsp. olive oil
» 4 garlic cloves, peeled
» 4 rosemary sprigs

Directions:

1. Take the fryer pan, place lamb chops in it, season the top with ½ tsp. black pepper and ¾ tsp. salt, then drizzle evenly with oil and spread with 1 tsp. minced garlic.
2. Add garlic cloves and rosemary and then let the lamb chops marinate in the pan into the refrigerator for a minimum of 1 hour.
3. Then switch on the air fryer, insert fryer pan, then shut with its lid, set the fryer at 360°F, and cook for 6 minutes.
4. Flip the lamb chops, season them with remaining salt and black pepper, add remaining minced garlic, and continue cooking for 6 minutes or until lamb chops are cooked.
5. When the air fryer beeps, open its lid, transfer lamb chops to a plate and serve.

Nutrition:

- Calories: 616
- Carbs: 1 g
- Fat: 28 g
- Protein: 83 g
- Fiber: 0.3 g

Chapter 9.

FISH & SEAFOOD RECIPES

56. COCONUT SHRIMP

Preparation Time: 9 minutes

Cooking Time: 8-10 minutes

Servings: 4

Ingredients:

» 1/2 cup pork rinds: ½ cup (Crushed)
» 4 cups jumbo shrimp: 4 cups. (deveined)
» 1/2 cup coconut flakes, preferably
» 2 eggs
» 1/2 cup coconut flour
» 1/2 inch any your choice oil for frying
» Freshly ground black pepper and kosher salt to taste

Dipping sauce:

» 2-3 tbsp. powdered sugar as a substitute
» 3 tbsp. mayonnaise
» 1/2 cup sour cream
» 1/4 tsp. coconut extract or to taste
» 3 tbsp. coconut cream
» 1/4 tsp. pineapple flavoring as much to taste.
» 3 tbsp. coconut flakes preferably unsweetened (optional)

Directions:
Sauce:

1. Mix all the ingredients into a tiny bowl for the dipping sauce (Pineapple flavor). Combine well and put in the fridge until ready to serve.
2. Shrimps:

3. Whip all eggs in a deep bowl and in a small shallow bowl; add the crushed pork rinds, coconut flour, sea salt, coconut flakes, and freshly ground black pepper.
4. Put the shrimp one by one in the mixed eggs for dipping, then in the coconut flour blend. Put them on a clean plate or put them on your air fryer's basket.
5. Place the shrimp battered in a single layer on your air fryer basket. Spritz the shrimp with oil and cook for 8 to 10 minutes at 360°F, flipping them through halfway.
6. Enjoy hot with dipping sauce.

Nutrition:

• Calories: 340
• Proteins: 25 g
• Carbs: 9 g
• Fat: 16 g

57. SALMON CAKES IN AIR FRYER

Preparation Time: 9 minutes

Cooking Time: 7 minutes

Servings: 2

Ingredients:

- » 8 oz. fresh salmon fillet
- » 1 egg
- » 1/8 salt
- » 1/4 garlic powder
- » 1 Sliced lemon

Directions:

1. In the bowl, chop the salmon, add the egg and spices.
2. Form tiny cakes.
3. Let the air fryer preheat to 390°F. On the bottom of the air fryer bowl lay sliced lemons—place cakes on top.
4. Cook them for 7 minutes. Based on your diet preferences, eat with your chosen dip.

Nutrition:

- Calories: 194
- Fat: 9 g
- Carbs: 1 g
- Proteins: 25 g

58. CRISPY FISH STICKS IN AIR FRYER

Preparation Time: 9 minutes

Cooking Time: 10 minutes

Servings: 4

Ingredients:

- » 1 lb. whitefish such as cod
- » 1/4 cup mayonnaise
- » 2 tbsp. Dijon mustard
- » 2 tbsp. water
- » 1 ½ cup pork rind
- » 3/4 tsp. Cajun seasoning
- » Kosher salt and pepper to taste
- » Cooking spray

Directions:

1. Spray with non-stick cooking spray to the air fryer rack.
2. Pat the fish dry and cut into sticks about 1 inch by 2 inches' broad
3. Stir together the mayonnaise, mustard, and water in a tiny small dish. Mix the pork rinds and Cajun seasoning into another small container.
4. Adding kosher salt and pepper to taste (both pork rinds and seasoning can have a decent amount of kosher salt, so you can dip a finger to see how salty it is).
5. Working for one slice of fish at a time, dip to cover in the mayonnaise mix, and then tap off the excess. Dip into the mixture of pork rind, then flip to cover. Place on the rack of an air fryer.
6. Set at 400°F to air fry for 5 minutes, then turn the fish with tongs and bake for another 5 minutes. Serve.

Nutrition:

- Calories: 263
- Fat: 16 g
- Carbs: 1 g
- Proteins: 26.4 g

59. HONEY-GLAZED SALMON

Preparation Time: 11 minutes

Cooking Time: 16 minutes

Servings: 2

Ingredients:

» 6 tsp. gluten-free soy sauce
» 2 pcs. Salmon fillets
» 3 tsp. sweet rice wine
» 1 tsp. water
» 6 tbsp. honey

Directions:

1. In a bowl, mix sweet rice wine, soy sauce, honey, and water.
2. Set half of it aside.
3. In half of it, marinate the fish and let it rest for 2 hours.
4. Let the air fryer preheat to 180°C.
5. Cook the fish for 8 minutes, flip halfway through, and cook for another 5 minutes.
6. Baste the salmon with marinade mixture after 3 or 4 minutes.
7. The half of marinade, pour in a saucepan, reduce to half, serve with a sauce.

Nutrition:

• Calories: 254
• Fat: 12 g
• Carbs: 9.9 g
• Proteins: 20 g

60. BASIL-PARMESAN CRUSTED SALMON

Preparation Time: 5 minutes

Cooking Time: 7 minutes

Servings: 4

Ingredients:

» 3 tbsp. grated Parmesan
» 4 skinless salmon fillets
» 1/4 tsp. salt
» Freshly ground black pepper
» 3 tbsp. low-fat mayonnaise
» ¼ cup basil leaves, chopped
» 1/2 lemon
» Olive oil for spraying

Directions:

1. Let the air fryer preheat to 400°F. Spray the basket with olive oil.
2. With salt, pepper, and lemon juice, season the salmon.
3. In a bowl, mix 2 tablespoons of Parmesan cheese with mayonnaise and basil leaves.
4. Add this mix and more parmesan on top of salmon and cook for 7 minutes or until fully cooked.
5. Serve hot.

Nutrition:

• Calories: 289
• Fat: 18.5 g
• Carbs: 1.5 g
• Proteins: 30 g

61. CAJUN SHRIMP IN AIR FRYER

Preparation Time: 9 minutes

Cooking Time: 3 minutes

Servings: 4

Ingredients:

» 24 extra-jumbo shrimp, peeled,
» 2 tbsp. olive oil
» 1 tbsp. Cajun seasoning
» 1 zucchini, thick slices (half-moons)
» 1/4 cup cooked turkey
» 2 yellow squash, sliced half-moons
» 1/4 tsp. kosher salt

Directions:

1. In a bowl, mix the shrimp with Cajun seasoning.
2. In another bowl, add zucchini, turkey, salt, squash, and coat with oil.
3. Let the air fryer preheat to 400°F.
4. Move the shrimp and vegetable mix to the fryer basket and cook for 3 minutes.
5. Serve hot.

Nutrition:

- Calories: 284
- Fat: 14 g
- Carbs: 8 g
- Proteins: 31 g

62. CRISPY AIR FRYER FISH

Preparation Time: 11 minutes

Cooking Time: 18 minutes

Servings: 4

Ingredients:

» 2 tsp. old bay
» 4–6, cut in half, whiting fish fillets
» 1/4 cup fine cornmeal
» 1/4 cup flour
» 1 tsp paprika
» 1/2 tsp. garlic powder
» 1 ½ tsp. salt
» ½ freshly ground black pepper

Directions:

1. In a Ziploc bag, add all ingredients and coat the fish fillets with it.
2. Spray oil on the basket of the air fryer and put the fish in it.
3. Cook for ten minutes at 400°F. Flip fish if necessary and coat with oil spray and cook for another 7 minutes.
4. Serve with salad green.

Nutrition:

- Calories: 254
- Fat: 12.7 g
- Carbs: 8.2 g
- Proteins: 17.5 g

63. AIR FRYER LEMON COD

Preparation Time: 5 minutes

Cooking Time: 10 minutes

Servings: 1

Ingredients:

- » 1 cod fillet
- » 1 tbsp. chopped dried parsley
- » Kosher salt and pepper to taste
- » 1 tbsp. garlic powder
- » 1 lemon

Directions:

1. In a bowl, mix all ingredients and coat the fish fillet with spices.
2. Slice the lemon and lay it at the bottom of the air fryer basket.
3. Put spiced fish on top. Cover the fish with lemon slices.
4. Cook for 10 minutes at 375°F, the internal temperature of fish should be 145°F.
5. Serve.

Nutrition:

- Calories: 101
- Fat: 1 g
- Carbs: 10 g
- Proteins: 16g

64. AIR FRYER SALMON FILLETS

Preparation Time: 5 minutes

Cooking Time: 15 minutes

Servings: 2

Ingredients:

- » 1/4 cup low-fat Greek yogurt
- » 2 salmon fillets
- » 1 tbsp. fresh dill (chopped)
- » 1 lemon juice
- » 1/2 garlic powder
- » Kosher salt and pepper

Directions:

1. Cut the lemon into slices and lay it at the bottom of the air fryer basket.
2. Season the salmon with kosher salt and pepper. Put salmon on top of lemons.
3. Let it cook at 330°F for 15 minutes.
4. In the meantime, mix garlic powder, lemon juice, salt, pepper with yogurt and dill.
5. Serve the fish with sauce.

Nutrition:

- Calories: 194
- Fat: 7 g
- Carbs: 6 g
- Proteins: 25 g

65. AIR FRYER FISH AND CHIPS

Preparation Time: 11 minutes

Cooking Time: 35 minutes

Servings: 4

Ingredients:

- » 4 cups any fish fillet
- » 1/4 cup flour
- » 1 cup whole-wheat breadcrumbs
- » 1 egg
- » 2 tbsp. oil
- » 2 potatoes
- » 1 tsp. salt

Directions:

1. Cut the potatoes in fries. Then coat with oil and salt.
2. Cook in the air fryer for 20 minutes at 400°F, toss the fries halfway through.
3. In the meantime, coat fish in flour, then in the whisked egg, and finally in breadcrumbs mix.
4. Place the fish in the air fryer and let it cook at 330°F for 15 minutes.
5. Flip it halfway through, if needed.
6. Serve with tartar sauce and salad green.

Nutrition:

- Calories: 409
- Fat: 11 g
- Carbs: 44 g
- Proteins: 30 g

66. GRILLED SALMON WITH LEMON

Preparation Time: 9 minutes

Cooking Time: 8 minutes

Servings: 4

Ingredients:

- » 2 tbsp. olive oil
- » 2 salmon fillets
- » 1/3 cup lemon juice
- » 1/3 cup water
- » 1/3 cup gluten-free light soy sauce
- » 1/3 cup honey
- » Scallion slices to garnish
- » Freshly ground black pepper, garlic powder, kosher salt to taste

Directions:

1. Season salmon with pepper and salt.
2. In a bowl, mix honey, soy sauce, lemon juice, water, oil. Add salmon to this marinade and let it rest for at least 2 hours.
3. Let the air fryer preheat at 180°C.
4. Place fish in the air fryer and cook for 8 minutes.
5. Move to a dish and top with scallion slices.

Nutrition:

- Calories: 211
- Fat: 9 g
- Carbs: 4.9 g
- Proteins: 15 g

67. AIR-FRIED FISH NUGGETS

Preparation Time: 15 minutes

Cooking Time: 12 minutes

Servings: 4

Ingredients:

- » 2 cups (skinless) fish fillets in cubes
- » 1 egg beaten
- » 5 tbsp. flour
- » 5 tbsp. water
- » Kosher salt and pepper to taste
- » ½ cup breadcrumbs mix
- » 1/4 cup whole-wheat breadcrumbs
- » Oil for spraying

Directions:

1. Season the fish cubes with kosher salt and pepper.
2. In a bowl, add flour and gradually add water, mixing as you add.
3. Then mix in the egg. And keep mixing but do not over mix.
4. Coat the cubes in batter, then in the breadcrumb mix. Coat well.
5. Place the cubes in a baking tray and spray with oil.
6. Let the air fryer preheat to 200°C.
7. Place cubes in the air fryer and cook for 12 minutes or until well cooked and golden brown.
8. Serve with salad greens.

Nutrition:

- Calories: 184
- Fat: 3 g
- Carbs: 10 g
- Proteins: 19 g

68. GARLIC ROSEMARY GRILLED PRAWNS

Preparation Time: 5 minutes

Cooking Time: 11 minutes

Servings: 2

Ingredients:

- » 1/2 tbsp. melted butter
- » 8 green capsicum slices
- » 8 prawns
- » 1/8 cup rosemary leaves
- » Kosher salt and freshly ground black pepper
- » 3-4 cloves minced garlic

Directions:

1. In a bowl, mix all the ingredients and marinate the prawns in it for at least 60 minutes or more.
2. Add 2 prawns and 2 slices of capsicum on each skewer.
3. Let the air fryer preheat to 180°C.
4. Cook for 5 to 6 minutes. Then change the temperature to 200°C and cook for another 5 minutes.
5. Serve with lemon wedges.

Nutrition:

- Calories: 194
- Fat: 10 g
- Carbs: 12 g
- Proteins: 26 g
-

Chapter 10.

VEGETARIAN RECIPES

69. CRISPY POTATOES AND PARSLEY

Preparation Time: 10 minutes

Cooking Time: 10 minutes

Servings: 4

Ingredients:

» 1-pound gold potatoes, cut into wedges
» Salt and black pepper to the taste
» 2tablespoons olive
» Juice from ½ lemon
» ¼ cup parsley leaves, chopped

Directions:

1. Rub potatoes with salt, pepper, lemon juice and olive oil, put them in your air fryer and cook at 350 degrees F for 10 minutes. Divide among plates, sprinkle parsley on top and serve. Enjoy!

Nutrition:

- Calories: 152
- Fat: 3
- Fiber :7
- Carbs: 17
- Protein: 4

70. CARROTS AND TURNIPS

Preparation Time: 10–20 minutes

Cooking Time: 9 minutes

Servings: 4

Ingredients:

» 2 turnips, peeled and sliced
» 1 small onion; chopped.
» 1 tsp. lemon juice
» 1 tsp. cumin, ground.
» 3 carrots, sliced
» 1 tbsp. extra-virgin olive oil
» 1 cup water
» Salt and black pepper to the taste

Directions:

1. Set your air fryer, add oil, and heat it.
2. Add onion, stir, and saute for 2 minutes.
3. Add turnips, carrots, cumin, and lemon juice, stir, and cook for 1 minute.
4. Add salt, pepper, and water, then stir well. Cook at high for 6 minutes.
5. Open the air fryer oven lid, and divide turnips and carrots among plates and serve.

Nutrition:

- Calories: 170
- Fat: 9 g
- Protein: 1 g
- Sugar: 5 g
- Carbs: 19 g
- Fiber: 7 g
- Sodium: 475 mg

71. INSTANT BRUSSELS SPROUTS WITH PARMESAN

Preparation Time: 10–20 minutes

Cooking Time: 3 minutes

Servings: 4

Ingredients:

- » 1 lb. brussels sprouts, washed
- » 1 cup water
- » 3 tbsp. Parmesan, grated
- » 1 lemon juice
- » 2 tbsp. butter
- » Salt and black pepper to taste

Directions:

1. Put sprouts in your air fryer oven, add salt, pepper, and water; and then stir well. Close the lid and cook at high for 3 minutes.
2. Transfer sprouts to a bowl, discard water and clean your air fryer.
3. Set your air fryer; add butter and melt it.
4. Add lemon juice and stir well.
5. Add sprouts, stir and transfer to plates.
6. Add more salt, pepper if needed, and Parmesan cheese on top.

Nutrition:

- Calories: 230
- Fat: 10 g
- Protein: 8 g
- Sugar: 5 g

72. BRAISED FENNEL

Preparation Time: 10–20 minutes

Cooking Time: 14 minutes

Servings: 4

Ingredients:

- » 2 fennel bulbs, trimmed and cut into quarters
- » 3 tbsp. extra-virgin olive oil
- » 1/4 cup white wine
- » 1/4 cup Parmesan, grated
- » 3/4 cup veggie stock
- » 1/2 lemon juice
- » 1 garlic clove; chopped.
- » 1 dried red pepper
- » Salt and black pepper to the taste

Directions:

1. Add oil and heat it.
2. Add garlic and red pepper, then stir well. Cook for 2 minutes and discard garlic.
3. Add fennel, stir and brown it for 8 minutes.
4. Add salt, pepper, stock, wine, close the lid and cook at high for 4 minutes.
5. Open the air fryer oven lid, add lemon juice, more salt and pepper if needed, and cheese.
6. Mix to coat, divide among plates and serve.

Nutrition:

- Calories: 230
- Fat: 4 g
- Protein: 1 g
- Sugar: 3 g
-

73. ROASTED POTATOES

Preparation Time: 10–20 minutes

Cooking Time: 17 minutes

Servings: 4

Ingredients:

» 2 lb. baby potatoes
» 5 tbsp. vegetable oil
» 1/2 cup stock
» 1 rosemary spring
» 5 garlic cloves
» Salt and black pepper to taste

Directions:

1. Set your air fryer oven on "Air Fryer" mode; add oil and heat it.
2. Add potatoes, rosemary and garlic, stir and brown them for 10 minutes.
3. Prick each potato with a knife, add the stock, salt, and pepper, seal the air fryer oven lid and cook at high for 7 minutes.
4. Open the air fryer, divide potatoes among plates and serve.

Nutrition:

- Calories: 250
- Fat: 15 g
- Protein: 2 g
- Sugar: 1 g

74. CREAMED SPINACH

Preparation Time: 10 minutes

Cooking Time: 20 minutes

Servings: 2

Ingredients:

» 1/2 cup chopped white onion
» 10 oz. frozen spinach, thawed
» 1 tsp. salt
» 1 tsp. ground black pepper
» 2 tsp. minced garlic
» 1/2 tsp. ground nutmeg
» 4 oz. cream cheese, reduced-fat, diced
» 1/4 cup shredded Parmesan cheese, reduced-fat
» 2 tbsp of olive oil

Directions:

1. Switch on the air fryer, insert fryer basket, grease it with olive oil, then shut with its lid, set the fryer at 350°F, and preheat for 5 minutes.
2. Meanwhile, take a 6-inches baking pan, grease it with oil, and set it aside.
3. Put spinach in a basin, add remaining ingredients except for Parmesan cheese, stir until well mixed and then add the mixture into a prepared baking pan.
4. Open the fryer, add pan in it, close with its lid and cook for 10 minutes until cooked and cheese has melted, stirring halfway through.
5. Then sprinkle Parmesan cheese on top of spinach and continue air frying for 5 minutes at 400°F until the top is nicely golden and cheese has melted.
6. Serve straight away.

Nutrition:

- Calories: 273
- Carbs: 8 g
- Fat: 23 g
- Protein: 8 g
- Fiber: 2 g

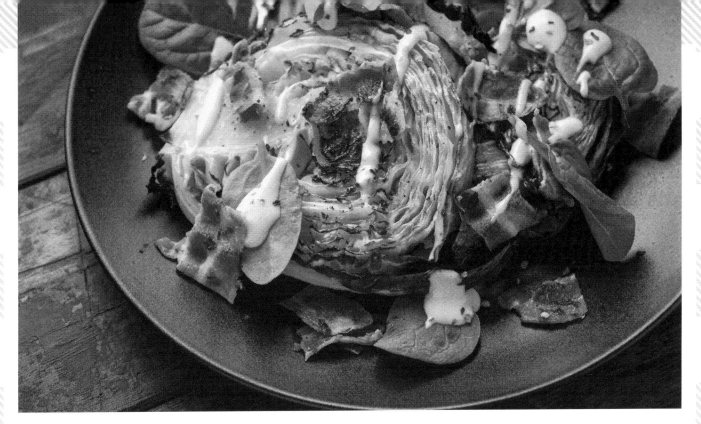

75. CABBAGE WEDGES

Preparation Time: 10 minutes

Cooking Time: 29 minutes

Servings: 2

Ingredients:

- » 1 small head green cabbage
- » 6 strips bacon, thick-cut, pastured
- » 1 tsp. onion powder
- » 1/2 tsp. ground black pepper
- » 1 tsp. garlic powder
- » 3/4 tsp. salt
- » 1/4 tsp. red chili flakes
- » 1/2 tsp. fennel seeds
- » 3 tbsp. olive oil

Directions:

1. Switch on the air fryer, insert fryer basket, grease it with olive oil, then shut with its lid, set the fryer to 350°F, and preheat for 5 minutes.
2. Open the fryer, add bacon strips in it, close with its lid and cook for 10 minutes until nicely golden and crispy, turning the bacon halfway through the frying.
3. Meanwhile, prepare the cabbage, remove the cabbage's outer leaves, and then cut it into 8 wedges, keeping the core intact.
4. Prepare the spice mix and for this, place onion powder in a bowl, add black pepper, garlic powder, salt, red chili, and fennel and stir until mixed.
5. Drizzle cabbage wedges with oil and then sprinkle with spice mix until well coated.
6. When the air fryer beeps, open its lid, transfer bacon strips to a cutting board and let it rest.
7. Add seasoned cabbage wedges into the fryer basket, close with its lid, then cook for 8 minutes at 400°F, flip the cabbage, spray with oil and continue air frying for 6 minutes until nicely golden and cooked.
8. When done, transfer cabbage wedges to a plate.
9. Chop the bacon, sprinkle it over cabbage and serve.

Nutrition:

- Calories: 123
- Carbs: 2 g
- Fat: 11 g
- Protein: 4 g
- Fiber: 0 g
- Sugar: 1 g

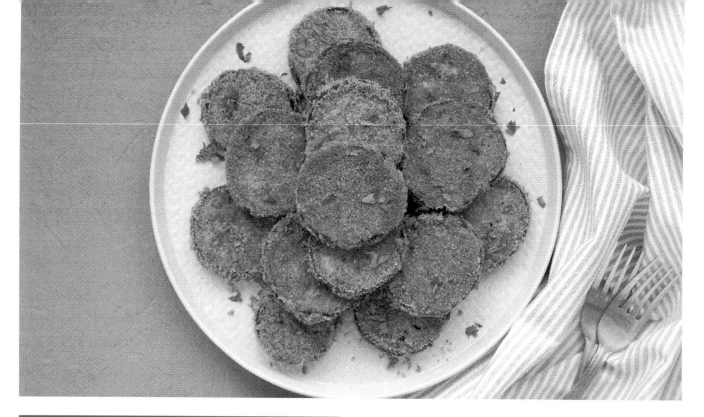

76. EGGPLANT PARMESAN

Preparation Time: 20 minutes

Cooking Time: 15 minutes

Servings: 4

Ingredients:

» 1/2 cup and 3 tbsp. almond flour, divided
» 1 ¼ lb. eggplant, ½-inch sliced
» 1 tbsp. chopped parsley
» 1 tsp. Italian seasoning
» 2 tsp. salt
» 1 cup marinara sauce
» 1 egg, pastured
» 1 tbsp. water
» 3 tbsp. grated Parmesan cheese, reduced-fat
» 1/4 cup grated mozzarella cheese, reduced-fat

Directions:

1. Slice the eggplant into ½-inch pieces, place them in a colander, sprinkle with 1 ½ teaspoon of salt on both sides, and let it rest for 15 minutes.
2. Meanwhile, place ½ cup flour in a bowl, add egg and water and whisk until blended.
3. Place remaining flour in a shallow dish, add remaining salt, Italian seasoning, and Parmesan cheese, and stir until mixed.

4. Switch on the air fryer, insert fryer basket, grease it with olive oil, then shut with its lid, set the fryer to 360°F, and preheat for 5 minutes.
5. Meanwhile, drain the eggplant pieces, pat them dry, and then dip each slice into the egg mixture and coat with flour mixture.
6. Open the air fryer, add coated eggplant slices in it in a single layer, close with its lid and cook for 8 minutes until nicely golden and cooked, flipping the eggplant slices halfway through the frying.
7. Then top each eggplant slice with a tbsp. of marinara sauce and some of the Mozzarella cheese and continue air frying for 1 to 2 minutes or until cheese has melted.
8. When the air fryer beeps, open its lid, transfer eggplants onto a serving plate, and keep them warm.
9. Cook the remaining eggplant slices the same way and serve.

Nutrition:

- Calories: 193
- Carbs: 27 g
- Fat: 5.5 g
- Protein: 10 g
- Fiber: 6 g

Chapter 11.
SNACKS RECIPES

77. SWEET POTATO FRIES

Preparation Time: 5 minutes

Cooking Time: 8 minutes

Servings: 4

Ingredients:

» 2 medium sweet potatoes, peeled
» 1 tbsp. arrowroot starch
» 2 tbsp. cinnamon
» 1/4 cup coconut sugar
» 2 tsp. melted butter, unsalted
» 1/2 tbsp. olive oil
» Confectioners swerve as needed

Directions:

1. Switch on the air fryer, insert fryer basket, grease it with olive oil, then shut with its lid, set the fryer to 370°F, and preheat for 5 minutes.
2. Meanwhile, cut peeled sweet potatoes into ½-inch thick slices, place them in a bowl, add oil and starch and toss until well coated.
3. Open the fryer, add sweet potatoes to it, close with its lid, and cook for 8 minutes until nicely golden, shaking halfway through the frying.
4. When the air fryer beeps, open its lid, transfer sweet potato fries in a bowl, add butter, sprinkle with sugar and cinnamon and toss until well mixed.
5. Sprinkle confectioners swerve on the fries and serve.

Nutrition:

- Calories: 130
- Carbs: 27 g
- Fat: 2.3 g
- Protein: 1.2 g
- Fiber: 3 g

78. CHEESE STICKS

Preparation Time: 5–7 minutes

Cooking Time: 5 minutes

Servings: 2

Ingredients:

» 10 pcs. spring roll wrappers, separated, quartered
» 1/4 lb. sharp cheddar cheese, reduced-fat, sliced into 2" x ½" matchsticks
» Oil for spraying

Directions:

1. Preheat the air fryer to 400°F.
2. Place cheese matchstick at the widest end of quartered spring roll wrapper. Moisten edges and tip of the wrapper with water. Fold spring roll wrapper over cheese, and tuck in both ends. Roll spring rolls tightly up to the tip. Place this into a freezer-safe container lined with saran wrap. Repeat the step for all cheese and spring roll wrappers.
3. Freeze for 1 hour before frying.
4. Spray a small amount of oil all over cheese matchsticks. Place a generous handful inside the air fryer basket. Fry for 3 to 5 minutes, or only until wrappers turn golden brown. Shake contents of the basket once midway through.
5. Remove from the basket. Set on plates. Repeat the step for the remaining breaded cheese sticks. Serve.

Nutrition:

• Calories: 229
• Carbs: 16 g
• Fat: 10 g
• Protein: 15 g
• Fiber: 1.0 g

79. ZUCCHINI CRISPS

Preparation Time: 30 minutes

Cooking Time: 30 minutes

Servings: 2

Ingredients:

» 2 zucchini, sliced into a 1/8-inch thick disk
» Pinch sea salt
» White pepper to taste
» 1 tbsp. of olive oil for drizzling

Directions:

1. Preheat the air fryer to 330°F.
2. Put zucchini in a bowl with salt. Let it sit in a colander to drain for 30 minutes.
3. Layer zucchini in a baking dish. Drizzle in oil. Season with pepper. Place baking dish in the air fryer basket. Cook for 30 minutes.
4. Adjust seasoning. Serve.

Nutrition:

• Calories: 15.2
• Carbs: 3.6 g
• Fat: 0.1 g
• Protein: 0.6 g
• Fiber: 1.3 g

80. TORTILLAS IN GREEN MANGO SALSA

Preparation Time: 30 minutes

Cooking Time: 10 minutes

Servings: 4

Ingredients:

Tortillas:
- » 4 pcs. corn tortillas
- » 1 tbsp. olive oil
- » 1/16 tsp. sea salt

Green mango salsa:
- » 1 green/unripe mango, minced
- » 1 red/ripe Roma tomato, preferably minced
- » 1 shallot, peeled, minced
- » 1 fresh jalapeno pepper, minced
- » 1/4 red bell pepper, minced
- » 4 tbsp. fresh cilantro, minced
- » 1/4 cup lime juice, freshly squeezed
- » 1/16 tsp. salt

Directions:

1. Preheat the air fryer to 400°F.
2. Mix lime juice and salt in a bowl. Stir until solids dissolve. Add the remaining salsa ingredients. Chill in the fridge for at least 30 minutes. Stir again just before using.
3. Lightly brush oil on both sides of tortillas. Cut these into large triangles.
4. Place a generous handful of sliced tortillas in the basket. Fry these for 10 minutes or until bread blisters and turns golden brown. Shake contents of the basket once midway through.
5. Place cooked pieces on a plate. Repeat step for remaining tortillas. Season with salt.
6. Place equal portions of crispy tortillas on plates. Serve with green mango and tomato salsa on the side.

Nutrition:

- Calories: 128
- Carbs: 8.6 g
- Fat: 3.6 g
- Protein: 2.7 g
- Fiber: 5.7 g

81. SKINNY PUMPKIN CHIPS

Preparation Time: 20 minutes

Cooking Time: 13 minutes

Servings: 2

Ingredients:

- » 1 lb. pumpkin, cut into sticks
- » 1 tbsp. coconut oil
- » 1/2 tsp. rosemary
- » 1/2 tsp. basil
- » Salt and ground black pepper to taste

Directions:

1. Start by preheating the air fryer to 395°F. Brush the pumpkin sticks with coconut oil; add the spices and toss to combine.
2. Cook for 13 minutes, shaking the basket halfway through the cooking time.
3. Serve with mayonnaise. Enjoy!

Nutrition:

- Calories: 118
- Fat; 14.7 g
- Carbs; 2.2 g
- Protein; 6.2 g
- Sugars: 7 g

82. AIR FRIED RIPE PLANTAINS

Preparation Time: 10 minutes

Cooking Time: 10 minutes

Servings: 2

Ingredients:

» 2 pcs. large ripe plantain, peeled, sliced into inch thick disks
» 1 tbsp. coconut butter, unsweetened

Directions:

1. Preheat the air fryer to 350°F.
2. Brush a small amount of coconut butter on all sides of plantain disks.
3. Place one even layer into the air fryer basket, making sure none overlap or touch. Fry plantains for 10 minutes.
4. Remove from the basket. Place on plates. Repeat step for all plantains.
5. While plantains are still warm. Serve.

Nutrition:

- Calories: 209
- Carbs: 29 g
- Fat: 8 g
- Protein: 2.9 g
- Fiber: 3.5 g

83. AIR FRIED PLANTAINS IN COCONUT SAUCE

Preparation Time: 10 minutes

Cooking Time: 10 minutes

Servings: 4

Ingredients:

» 6 ripe plantains, peeled, quartered lengthwise
» 1 can coconut cream
» 2 tbsp. of honey
» 1 tbsp. of coconut oil

Directions:

1. Preheat the air fryer to 330°F.
2. Pour coconut cream in a thick-bottomed saucepan set over high heat; bring to boil. Reduce heat to lowest setting; simmer uncovered until the cream is reduced by half and darkens in color. Turn off heat.
3. Whisk in honey until smooth. Cool completely before using. Lightly grease a non-stick skillet with coconut oil.
4. Layer plantains in the air fryer basket and fry for 10 minutes or until golden on both sides; drain on paper towels. Place plantain on plates.
5. Drizzle in a small amount of coconut sauce. Serve.

Nutrition:

- Calories: 236
- Carbs: 0 g
- Fiber: 1.8 g
- Fat: 1.5 g
- Protein: 1 g

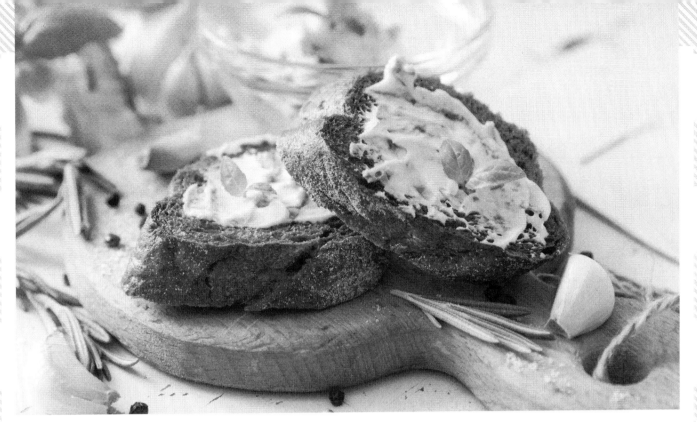

84. GARLIC BREAD WITH CHEESE DIP

Preparation Time: 10 minutes

Cooking Time: 5 minutes

Servings: 4

Ingredients:

» Fried garlic bread
» 1 medium baguette, halved lengthwise, cut sides toasted
» 2 garlic cloves, whole
» 4 tbsp. extra-virgin olive oil
» 2 tbsp. fresh parsley, minced
» Blue cheese dip:
» 1 tbsp. fresh parsley, minced
» 1/4 cup fresh chives, minced
» 1/4 tsp. Tabasco sauce
» 1 tbsp. lemon juice, freshly squeezed
» 1/2 cup Greek yogurt, low fat
» 1/4 cup blue cheese, reduced fat
» 1/16 tsp. salt
» 1/16 tsp. white pepper

Directions:

1. Preheat the machine to 400°F.
2. Mix oil and parsley in a small bowl.
3. Vigorously rub garlic cloves on cut/toasted sides of the baguette. Dispose of garlic nubs.
4. Using a pastry brush, spread parsley-infused oil on the cut side of the bread.
5. Place the bread cut-side down on a chopping board. Slice into inch-thick half-moons.
6. Place bread slices in an air fryer basket. Fry for 3 to 5 minutes or until bread browns a little. Shake contents of the basket once midway through. Place cooked pieces on a serving platter. Repeat the step for the remaining bread.
7. To prepare blue cheese dip, mix all the ingredients in a bowl.
8. Place equal portions of fried bread on plates. Serve with blue cheese dip on the side.

Nutrition:

• Calories: 209
• Carbs: 29 g
• Fat: 8 g
• Protein: 2.9 g
• Fiber: 3.5 g

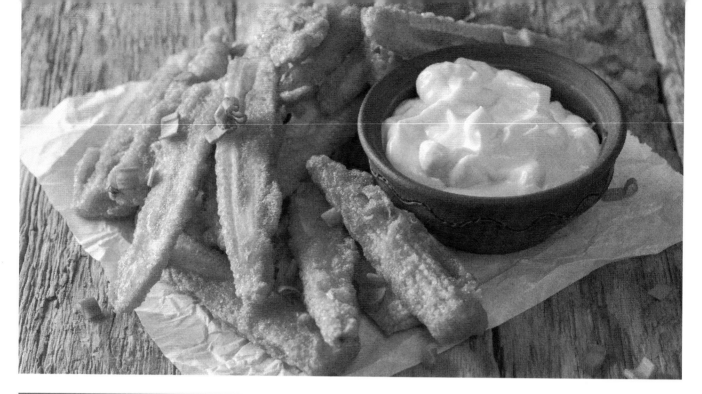

85. FRIED MIXED VEGGIES WITH AVOCADO DIP

Preparation Time: 10 minutes

Cooking Time: 10 minutes

Servings: 4

Ingredients:

- » Oil for spraying
- » 1 cup panko breadcrumbs. Add more if needed
- » 1 large egg, whisked, add more if needed
- » 1 cup all-purpose flour, add more if needed
- » 1/8 tsp. flaky sea salt
- » **Avocado-feta dip:**
- » 1 avocado, pitted, peeled, flesh scooped out
- » 4 oz. feta cheese, reduced fat
- » 2 leeks, minced
- » 1 lime, freshly squeezed
- » 1/4 cup fresh parsley, chopped roughly
- » 1/16 tsp. black pepper
- » 1/16 tsp. salt
- » **Vegetables:**
- » 1 zucchini, sliced into matchsticks
- » 1 carrot, sliced into matchsticks
- » 1 parsnip, sliced into matchsticks

Directions:

1. Preheat the air fryer to 400°F.
2. Season carrots, parsnips, and zucchini with salt.
3. Dredge carrots with flour first, then dip them into the whisked egg, and finally into breadcrumbs. Place breaded pieces on a baking sheet lined with parchment paper. Repeat the step for all carrots. Then do the same for parsnips and zucchini.
4. Lightly spray vegetables with oil. Place a generous handful of carrots in the air fryer basket. Fry for 10 minutes or until breading turns golden brown, shaking contents of the basket once midway. Place cooked pieces on a plate. Repeat the step for the remaining carrots.
5. Do the preceding step for parsnips and then zucchini.
6. For the dip, except for salt, place the remaining ingredients in a food processor. Pulse a couple of times, and then process to desired consistency scraping downsides of the machine often. Taste. Add salt only if needed. Place in an airtight container. Chill until needed.
7. Place equal portions of cooked vegetables on plates. Serve with a small amount of avocado-feta dip on the side.

Nutrition:

- Calories: 109
- Carbs: 4.0 g
- Fat: 2.6 g
- Protein: 2.9 g
- Fiber: 2.5 g

86. BEEF AND MANGO SKEWERS

Preparation Time: 10 minutes

Cooking Time: 4–7 minutes

Servings: 4

Ingredients:

» 3/4 lb. (340 g) of beef sirloin tip, cut into 1-inch cubes
» 2 tbsp. balsamic vinegar
» 1 tbsp. olive oil
» 1 tbsp. honey
» 1/2 tsp. dried marjoram
» Pinch salt
» Freshly ground black pepper to taste
» 1 mango

Directions:

1. Put the beef cubes in a medium bowl and add the balsamic vinegar, olive oil, honey, marjoram, salt, and pepper. Mix well, then rub the marinade into the beef with your hands. Set aside.
2. To prepare the mango, stand it on end and cut the skin off using a sharp knife. Then carefully cut around the oval pit to remove the flesh. Cut the mango into 1-inch cubes.
3. Thread metal skewers alternating with 3 beef cubes and 2 mango cubes. Place the skewers in the air fryer basket.
4. Air fry at 390°F (199°C) for 4 to 7 minutes or until the beef is browned and at least 145°F (63°C).

Nutrition:

- Calories: 245
- Fat: 9 g
- Protein: 26 g
- Carbs: 15 g
- Fiber: 1 g
- Sugar: 14 g
- Sodium: 96 mg

87. KALE CHIPS WITH LEMON YOGURT SAUCE

Preparation Time: 10 minutes

Cooking Time: 5 minutes

Servings: 4

Ingredients:

» 1 cup plain Greek yogurt
» 3 tbsp. freshly squeezed lemon juice
» 2 tbsp. honey mustard
» 1/2 tsp. dried oregano
» 1 bunch curly kale
» 2 tbsp. olive oil
» 1/2 tsp. salt
» 1/8 tsp. pepper

Directions:

1. In a small bowl, mix the yogurt, lemon juice, honey mustard, and oregano, and set aside.
2. Remove the stems and ribs from the kale with a sharp knife. Cut the leaves into 2 to 3-inch pieces.
3. Toss the kale with olive oil, salt, and pepper. Rub the oil into the leaves with your hands.
4. Air fry the kale in batches at 390°F (199°C) until crisp, about 5 minutes, shaking the basket once during cooking time. Serve with the yogurt sauce.

Nutrition:

- Calories: 155
- Fat: 8 g
- Protein: 8 g
- Carbs: 13 g
- Fiber: 1 g
- Sugar: 3 g
- Sodium: 378 mg

88. BASIL PESTO BRUSCHETTA

Preparation Time: 10 minutes

Cooking Time: 4–8 minutes

Servings: 4

Ingredients:

- » 8 slices French bread, ½-inch thick
- » 2 tbsp. softened butter
- » 1 cup shredded Mozzarella cheese
- » 1/2 cup basil pesto
- » 1 cup chopped grape tomatoes
- » 2 green onions, thinly sliced

Directions:

1. Spread the bread with the butter and place butter-side up in the air fryer basket. Bake at 350°F (177°C) for 3 to 5 minutes or until the bread is light golden brown.
2. Remove the bread from the basket and top each piece with some of the cheese. Return to the basket in batches and bake until the cheese melts for about 1 to 3 minutes.
3. Meanwhile, combine the pesto, tomatoes, and green onions in a small bowl.
4. When the cheese has melted, remove the bread from the air fryer and place it on a serving plate. Top each slice with some of the pesto mixture and serve.

Nutrition:

- Calories: 463
- Fat: 25 g
- Protein: 19 g
- Carbs: 41 g
- Fiber: 3 g
- Sugar: 2 g
- Sodium: 822 mg

89. CINNAMON PEAR CHIPS

Preparation Time: 15 minutes

Cooking Time: 9–13 minutes

Servings: 4

Ingredients:

- » 2 firm Bosc pears, cut crosswise into 1/8-inch thick slices
- » 1 tbsp. freshly squeezed lemon juice
- » 1/2 tsp. ground cinnamon
- » 1/8 tsp. ground cardamom or ground nutmeg

Directions:

1. Separate the smaller stem-end pear rounds from the larger rounds with seeds. Remove the core and seeds from the larger slices. Sprinkle all slices with lemon juice, cinnamon, and cardamom.
2. Put the smaller chips into the basket. Air fry at 380°F (193°C) for 3 to 5 minutes, until light golden brown, shaking the basket once during cooking. Remove from the air fryer.
3. Repeat with the larger slices, air frying for 6 to 8 minutes, until light golden brown, shaking the basket once during cooking.
4. Remove the chips from the air fryer. Cool and serve or store in an airtight container at room temperature for up to 2 days.

Nutrition:

- Calories: 31
- Fat: 0 g
- Protein: 7 g
- Carbs: 8 g
- Fiber: 2 g
- Sugar: 5 g
- Sodium: 0 mg

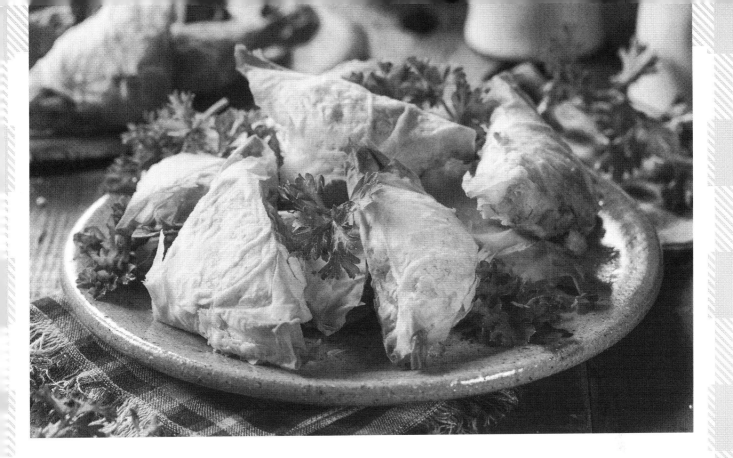

90. PHYLLO VEGETABLE TRIANGLES

Preparation Time: 15 minutes

Cooking Time: 6–11 minutes

Servings: 2

Ingredients:

- » 3 tbsp. minced onion
- » 2 garlic cloves, minced
- » 2 tbsp. grated carrot
- » 1 tsp. olive oil
- » 3 tbsp. frozen baby peas, thawed
- » 2 tbsp. non-fat cream cheese, at room temperature
- » 6 sheets frozen phyllo dough, thawed
- » Olive oil spray for coating the dough

Directions:

1. In a baking pan, combine the onion, garlic, carrot, and olive oil. Air fry at 390°F (199°C) for 2 to 4 minutes, or until the vegetables are crisp-tender. Transfer to a bowl.
2. Stir in the peas and cream cheese to the vegetable mixture. Let it cool while you prepare the dough.
3. Lay one sheet of phyllo on a work surface and lightly spray with olive oil spray. Top with another sheet of phyllo. Repeat with the remaining 4 phyllo sheets; you'll have 3 stacks with 2 layers each. Cut each stack lengthwise into 4 strips (12 strips total).
4. Place a scant 2 tsp. of the filling near the bottom of each strip. Bring one corner up over the filling to make a triangle; continue folding the triangles over, as you would fold a flag. Seal the edge with a bit of water. Repeat with the remaining strips and filling.
5. Air fry the triangles, in 2 batches, for 4 to 7 minutes or until golden brown. Serve.

Nutrition:

- • Calories: 67
- • Fat: 2 g
- • Protein: 2 g
- • Carbs: 11 g
- • Fiber: 1 g
- • Sugar: 1 g
- • Sodium: 121 mg
- •

Chapter 12.

DESSERTS RECIPES

91. BANANA BREAD

Preparation time: 5 minutes

Preparation time: 40 minutes

Servings: 6

Ingredients:

- » ¾ cup sugar
- » 1/3 cup butter
- » 1 tablespoon vanilla extract
- » 1 egg
- » 2 bananas
- » 1 tablespoon baking powder
- » 1 and ½ cups flour
- » ½ tablespoon baking soda
- » 1/3 cup milk
- » 1 and ½ tablespoon cream of tartar
- » Cooking spray

Directions:

1. Mix in milk with cream of tartar, vanilla, egg, sugar, bananas and butter in a bowl until well combined.
2. Mix in flour with baking soda and baking powder.
3. Blend the 2 mixtures, mix properly, move into pan greased with cooking spray, put into air fryer and cook at 320°F for 40 minutes.
4. Remove bread, allow to cool, slice.
5. Serve.

Nutrition:

- Calories: 540
- Total Fat: 16 grams
- Total Carbohydrate: 28 grams

92. SPECIAL BROWNIES

Preparation time: 10 minutes

Preparation time: 22 minutes

Servings: 4

Ingredients:

- » 1 egg
- » 1/3 cup cocoa powder
- » 1/3 cup sugar
- » 7 tablespoon butter
- » ½ tablespoon vanilla extract
- » ¼ cup white flour
- » ¼ cup walnuts
- » ½ tablespoon baking powder
- » 1 tablespoon peanut butter

Directions:

1. Warm pan with 6 tablespoons butter and the sugar over medium heat, cook for 5 minutes, transfer to a bowl, put salt, egg, cocoa powder, vanilla extract, walnuts, baking powder and flour, turn mix properly and into a pan.
2. Mix peanut butter with one tablespoon of butter in a bowl, heat in the microwave for some seconds, turn properly and sprinkle brownies blend over.
3. Put in air fryer and bake at 320° F and bake for 17 minutes.
4. Allow brownies to cool, cut.
5. Serve.

Nutrition:

- Calories: 230
- Fat: 10.1 g
- Carbs: 25 g
- Sugar: 16.7 g
- Protein: 9.2 g
- Cholesterol: 135 mg

93. CRISPY APPLES

Preparation time: 10 minutes

Preparation time: 10 minutes

Servings: 4

Ingredients:

- » 2 tablespoon cinnamon powder
- » 5 apples
- » 1 tablespoon maple syrup
- » ½ cup water
- » 4 tablespoon butter
- » ¼ cup flour
- » ¾ cup oats
- » ¼ cup brown sugar

Directions:

1. Cut the apples and put them in a pan, add in nutmeg, maple syrup, cinnamon and water.
2. Mix in butter with flour, sugar, salt and oat, turn, put spoonful of blend over apples, get into air fryer and cook at 350°F for 10 minutes.
3. Serve warm.

Nutrition:

- Calories: 387
- Total Fat: 5.6 grams
- Total Carbohydrate: 12.4 grams

94. COCONUT DONUTS

Preparation time: 5 minutes

Preparation time: 15 minutes

Servings: 4

Ingredients:

» 8 ounces coconut flour
» 1 egg, whisked
» 1 and ½ tablespoons butter, melted
» 4 ounces coconut milk
» 1 teaspoon baking powder

Directions:

1. In a bowl, put all of the ingredients and mix well.
2. Shape donuts from this mix, place them in your air fryer's basket and cook at 370 degrees F for 15 minutes.
3. Serve warm.

Nutrition:

- Calories :190
- Protein : 6 g.
- Fat :12 g.
- Carbs : 4 g.

95. BLUEBERRY CREAM

Preparation time: 4 minutes

Preparation time: 20 minutes

Servings: 6

Ingredients:

» 2 cups blueberries
» Juice of ½ lemon
» 2 tablespoons water
» 1 teaspoon vanilla extract
» 2 tablespoons swerve

Directions:

1. In a large bowl, put all ingredients and mix well.
2. Divide into 6 ramekins, put them in the air fryer and cook at 340 degrees F for 20 minutes
3. Cool down and serve.

Nutrition:

- Calories : 123
- Protein : 3 g.
- Fat : 2 g.
- Carbs : 4 g.

96. DONUTS

Preparation time: 10 minutes

Preparation time: 120 minutes

Servings: 14 donuts

Ingredients:

- » 3 cups of all-purpose flour
- » 1 cup of milk, warmed to around 110°F
- » 4 tablespoons of unsalted melted butter
- » 1 large egg
- » ¼ cup +1 teaspoon of sugar
- » 2 ½ teaspoons of active dry yeast
- » ½ teaspoon of kosher salt

For Glaze:

- » 2 cups of powdered sugar
- » 6 tablespoons of unsalted melted butter
- » 2 teaspoons of vanilla extract
- » 2–4 tablespoons of hot water

Directions:

1. Add the warm milk, yeast, and 1 teaspoon of sugar to a large bowl. Stir it for 5–10 minutes until foamy.
2. Add the egg, ¼ cup of sugar, and salt into the milk mixture. Stir it until combined. Pour in the melted butter with 2 cups of flour and mix.
3. Scrape the sides of the bowl down, and add in 1 more cup of flour. Mix it well until the dough starts pulling away from the bowl but leaves sticky. Continue kneading for 5–10 minutes. Cover the bowl with plastic wrap. Leave it for 30 minutes until the dough doubled.
4. Spread some flour on the work surface. Transfer the dough onto it and roll into a ½-¼-inch-thick layer. Cut out donuts with a round cutter (about 3 inches in diameter). Use a smaller cutter (about 1 inch in diameter) and cut out the centers.
5. Transfer the formed donuts onto the oiled parchment paper, and cover them with oiled plastic wrap. Leave it for 20–30 minutes until the dough is doubled.
6. Preheat your air fryer to 350°F. Spray the inside of the basket with some oil.
7. Put the formed donuts in the preheated air fryer in a single layer. Avoid them touching. Lightly spray tops with oil. Cook at 350°F for 4–5 minutes. Repeat this step with the remaining part of donuts and their holes.
8. For making glaze: Meantime, pour the melted butter into a medium bowl. Add in vanilla and powdered sugar. Whisk until combined. Stir in 1 tablespoon of hot water at a time until you reach the desired consistency.
9. After cooling the donuts for a few minutes, glaze them until fully coated. Put donuts on the rack to drip off the excess of the glaze until it hardens.
10. Serve and enjoy your Donuts!

Nutrition

- Calories: 270
- Carbohydrates: 32 g
- Fat: 14 g
- Protein: 3 g

- Sugar: 17 g
- Sodium: 70 g
- Cholesterol: 25 g

97. NUTTY MIX

Preparation time: 5 minutes

Preparation time: 4 minutes

Servings: 6

Ingredients:

- » 2 cup mix nuts
- » 1 tsp. ground cumin
- » 1 tsp. chili powder
- » 1 tbsp. melted butter
- » 1 tsp. salt
- » 1 tsp. pepper

Directions

1. Set all ingredients in a large bowl and toss until well coated.
2. Preheat the air fryer at 350 °F for 5 minutes.
3. Add mix nuts in air fryer basket and air fry for 4 minutes. Shake basket halfway through.
4. Serve and enjoy.

Nutrition:

- Calories: 316
- Fat :29g
- Carbohydrates: 11.3g
- Protein: 7.6g

98. CHOCOLATE CUP CAKES

Preparation time: 5 minutes

Preparation time: 12 minutes

Servings: 6

Ingredients:

- » 3 eggs
- » ¼ cup caster sugar
- » ¼ cup cocoa powder
- » 1 tsp. baking powder
- » 1 cup milk
- » ¼ tsp. vanilla essence
- » 2 cup all-purpose flour
- » 4 tbsps. Butter

Directions

1. Preheat your Air Fryer to a temperature of 400 °F (200 degrees Celsius).
2. Beat eggs with sugar in a bowl until creamy.
3. Add butter and beat again for 1-2 minutes.
4. Now add flour, cocoa powder, milk, and baking powder, and vanilla essence, mix with a spatula.
5. Fill ¾ of muffin tins with the mixture and place them into Air Fryer basket.
6. Let cook for 12 minutes.
7. Serve!

Nutrition:

- Calories 289
- Fat 11.5g
- Carbohydrates 38.94g
- Protein 8 7?g

99. VANILLA SPICED SOUFFLÉ

Preparation time: 20 minutes

Preparation time: 32 minutes

Servings: 6

Ingredients:

» ¼ cup all-purpose flour
» 1 cup whole milk
» 2 tsp. Vanilla extract
» 1 tsp. cream of tartar
» 1 vanilla bean
» 4 egg yolks
» 1-oz. sugar
» ¼ cup softened butter
» ¼ cup sugar
» 5 egg whites

Directions

1. Combine flour and butter in a bowl until the mixture becomes a smooth paste.
2. Set the pan over medium flame to heat the milk. Add sugar and stir until dissolved.
3. Mix in the vanilla bean and bring to a boil.
4. Beat the mixture using a wire whisk as you add the butter and flour mixture.
5. Lower the heat to simmer until thick. Discard the vanilla bean. Turn off the heat.
6. Place them on an ice bath and allow to cool for 10 minutes.
7. Grease 6 ramekins with butter. Sprinkle each with a bit of sugar.
8. Beat the egg yolks in a bowl. Add the vanilla extract and milk mixture. Mix until combined.
9. Whisk together the tartar cream, egg whites, and sugar until it forms medium stiff peaks.
10. Gradually fold egg whites into the soufflé base. Transfer the mixture to the ramekins.
11. Put 3 ramekins in the cooking basket at a time. Cook for 16 minutes at 330 degrees Fahrenheit. Move to a wire rack for cooling and cook the rest.
12. Sprinkle powdered sugar on top and drizzle with chocolate sauce before serving.

Nutrition:

- Calories 215
- Fat 12.2g
- Carbohydrates 18.98g
- Protein 6.66g

100. LATE CUP CAKES

Preparation time: 5 minutes

Preparation time: 12 minutes

Servings: 6

Ingredients:

- » 3 eggs
- » ¼ cup caster sugar
- » ¼ cup cocoa powder
- » 1 tsp. baking powder
- » 1 cup milk
- » ¼ tsp. vanilla essence
- » 2 cup all-purpose flour
- » 4 tbsps. Butter

Directions

1. Preheat your Air Fryer to a temperature of 400 °F (200 degrees Celsius).
2. Beat eggs with sugar in a bowl until creamy.
3. Add butter and beat again for 1-2 minutes.
4. Now add flour, cocoa powder, milk, and baking powder, and vanilla essence, mix with a spatula.
5. Fill ¾ of muffin tins with the mixture and place them into Air Fryer basket.
6. Let cook for 12 minutes.
7. Serve!

Nutrition:

- Calories 289
- Fat 11.5g
- Carbohydrates 38.94g
- Protein 8.72g

101. BLUEBERRY MUFFINS

Preparation time: 10 minutes

Preparation time: 35 minutes

Servings: 3

Ingredients

- » 1 egg
- » 2/3 cup of flour
- » ½ cup of blueberries*
- » 1/3 cup of oil
- » 1/3 cup of sugar
- » 2 tablespoons of water
- » 1 teaspoon of lemon zest
- » ½ teaspoon of baking powder
- » ¼ teaspoon of vanilla extract
- » Pinch of salt

Directions:

1. Preheat your air fryer to 350°F.
2. Add the egg, oil, water, and vanilla in a medium bowl. Whisk until smooth consistency.
3. Mix the sugar, lemon zest, flour, baking powder, and salt in a separate bowl. Add the dry ingredients into the wet ones. Stir until smooth.
4. Gently fold in the blueberries.
5. Cover oven-safe 1-cup ramekins with muffin papers. Put the prepared batter into each ramekin. Cook at 350°F for 15–17 minutes.
6. Serve and enjoy your Blueberry Muffins!

Nutrition

- Calories: 39
- Carbohydrates: 1 g
- Fat: 3 g
- Protein: 2 g
- Sugar: 1 g
- Sodium: 6,8 g
- Cholesterol: 6,2 gg

102. CHEESECAKE

Preparation time: 20 minutes

Preparation time: 20 minutes

Servings: 8-12

Ingredients:

- Crust
- 1/2 cup dates, chopped, soaked in water for at least 15 min., soaking liquid reserved
- 1/2 cup walnuts
- 1 cup quick oats

Filling

- 1/2 cup vanilla almond milk
- 1/4 cup coconut palm sugar
- 1/2 cup coconut flour
- 1 cup cashews, soaked in water for at least 2 hours
- 1 tsp. vanilla extract
- 2 tbsp. lemon juice
- 1 to 2 tsp. grated lemon zest
- 1/2 cup fresh berries or 6 figs, sliced
- 1 tbsp. arrowroot powder

Directions:

1. Make the crust: in a food processor, process together all the crust ingredients until smooth and press the mixture into the bottom of a spring form pan.
2. Make the filling: add cashews along with soaking liquid to a blender and process until very smooth; add milk, palm sugar, coconut flour, lemon juice, lemon zest, and vanilla and blend until well combined; add arrowroot and continue blending until mixed and pour into the crust. Smooth the top and cover the spring form pan with foil.
3. Place the pan in your air fry toaster oven and bake at 375 °F for 20 minutes.
4. Carefully remove the pan from the fryer and remove the foil; let the cake cool completely and top with fruit to serve.

Nutrition:

- Calories 423
- Fat 3.1g
- Carbohydrates 33.5g
- Protein 1.2g

103. STRAWBERRY PIE

Preparation time: 10 minutes

Preparation time: 20 minutes

Servings: 12

Ingredients:

For the crust:
- » 1 cup coconut, shredded
- » 1 cup sunflower seeds
- » ¼ cup butter

For the filling:
- » 1 teaspoon gelatin
- » 8 ounces cream cheese
- » 4 ounces strawberries
- » 2 tablespoons water
- » ½ tablespoon lemon juice
- » ¼ teaspoon stevia
- » ½ cup heavy cream
- » 8 ounces strawberries, chopped for serving

Directions:

1. In your food processor, mix sunflower seeds with coconut, a pinch of salt and butter, pulse and press this on the bottom of a cake pan that fits your Air Fryer.
2. Heat up a pan with the water over medium heat, add gelatin, stir until it dissolves; leave aside to cool down. Add this to your food processor, mix with 4 ounces strawberries, cream cheese, lemon juice and stevia and blend well.
3. Add heavy cream, stir well and spread this over crust.
4. Top with 8 ounces strawberries, introduce in your Air Fryer and cook at 330 degrees F for 15 minutes.
5. Keep in the fridge until you serve it. Enjoy!

Nutrition:
- Calories 234
- Fat 23 g
- Fiber 2 g
- Carbs 6 g
- Protein 7 g

104. MINI LAVA CAKES

Preparation time: 10 minutes

Preparation time: 20 minutes

Servings: 3

Ingredients:

- » 1 egg
- » 4 tablespoons sugar
- » 2 tablespoons olive oil
- » 4 tablespoons milk
- » 4 tablespoons flour
- » 1 tablespoon cocoa powder
- » ½ teaspoon baking powder
- » ½ teaspoon orange zest

Directions:

1. In a bowl, mix egg with sugar, oil, milk, flour, salt, cocoa powder, baking powder and orange zest, stir very well and pour this into greased ramekins.
2. Add ramekins to your Air Fryer and cook at 320 degrees F for 20 minutes.
3. Serve lava cakes warm. Enjoy!

Nutrition:
- Calories 201
- Fat 7
- Fiber 8
- Carbs 23
- Protein 4

105. BERRY CRUMBLE

Preparation time: 10 Minutes

Preparation time: 15 minutes

Servings: 6

Ingredients:

For the Filling:
- »   2 cups mixed berries
- »   2 tablespoons sugar
- »   1tablespoon cornstarch
- »   1tablespoon fresh lemon juice

For the Topping:
- »   ¼ cup rolled oats
- »   1tablespoon sugar
- »   1tbsp. Whipped cream or ice cream (optional)

Directions:

1. Preheat the air fryer to 400°F (204°C).
2. For the filling: in a round baking pan, gently mix the berries, sugar, cornstarch, and lemon juice until thoroughly combined.
3. For the topping: in a small bowl, combine the flour, oats, and sugar. Stir the butter into the flour mixture until the mixture has the consistency of bread crumbs.
4. Sprinkle the topping over the berries.
5. Put the pan in the air fryer basket and air fry for 15 minutes. Let cool for 5 minutes on a wire rack.
6. Serve topped with whipped cream or ice cream, if desired.

Nutrition:
- Calories 123 kcal
- Fat 1 g
- Carbs 2 g
- Protein 4 g

Chapter 13.
30 DAY MEAL PLAN

Day	Lunch	Dinner	Desserts/Snacks
1	Salmon Cakes in Air Fryer	Duo Crisp Chicken Wings	Banana Bread
2	Coconut Shrimp	Crispy Potatoes And Parsley	Special Brownies
3	Crispy Fish Sticks in Air Fryer	Chicken Pot Pie	Crispy Apples
4	Honey-Glazed Salmon	Chicken Casserole	Coconut Donuts
5	Basil-Parmesan Crusted Salmon	Ranch Chicken Wings	Blueberry Cream
6	Cajun Shrimp in Air Fryer	Chicken Mac and Cheese	Nutty Mix
7	Crispy Air Fryer Fish	Broccoli Chicken Casserole	Donuts
8	Air Fryer Lemon Cod	Chicken Tikka Kebab	Vanilla Spiced Soufflé
9	Air Fryer Salmon Fillets	Bacon-Wrapped Chicken	Chocolate Cup Cakes

9	Air Fryer Salmon Fillets	Bacon-Wrapped Chicken	Chocolate Cup Cakes
10	Air Fryer Fish and Chips	Creamy Chicken Thighs	Cheesecake
11	Grilled Salmon with Lemon	Air Fryer Teriyaki Hen Drumsticks	Blueberry Muffins
12	Air-Fried Fish Nuggets	Duo Crisp Chicken Wings	Strawberry Pie
13	Garlic Rosemary Grilled Prawns	Crispy Potatoes And Parsley	Mini Lava Cakes
14	Salmon Cakes in Air Fryer	Chicken Pot Pie	Berry Crumble
15	Coconut Shrimp	Chicken Casserole	Banana Bread
16	Greek Lamb Pita Pockets	Meatloaf Slider Wraps	Sweet Potato Fries
17	Rosemary Lamb Chops	Double Cheeseburger	Cheese Sticks
18	Herb Butter Lamb Chops	Beef Schnitzel	Zucchini Crisps

19	Za'atar Lamb Chops	Steak with Asparagus Bundles	Tortillas in Green Mango Salsa
20	Greek Lamb Chops	Hamburgers	Air Fried Ripe Plantains
21	Herbed Lamb Chops	Beef Steak Kabobs with Vegetables	Garlic Bread with Cheese Dip
22	Spicy Lamb Sirloin Steak	Rib-Eye Steak	Fried Mixed Veggies with Avocado Dip
23	Garlic Rosemary Lamb Chops	Bunless Sloppy Joes	Air Fried Plantains in Coconut Sauce
24	Cherry-Glazed Lamb Chops	Beef Curry	Beef and Mango Skewers
25	Lamb and Vegetable Stew	Asian Grilled Beef Salad	Kale Chips with Lemon Yogurt Sauce
26	Lime Parsley Lamb Cutlets	Sunday Pot Roast	Sweet Potato Fries
27	Greek Lamb Pita Pockets	Beef Burrito Bowl	Cheese Sticks

28	Rosemary Lamb Chops	Beef and Pepper Fajita Bowls	Zucchini Crisps
29	Herb Butter Lamb Chops	Meatloaf Slider Wraps	Tortillas in Green Mango Salsa
30	Za'atar Lamb Chops	Double Cheeseburger	Air Fried Ripe Plantains

Chapter 14

MEASUREMENT CONVERSIONS

VOLUME EQUIVALENTS(DRY)

US STANDARD	METRIC (APPROXIMATE)
1/8 teaspoon	0.5 mL
1/4 teaspoon	1 mL
1/2 teaspoon	2 mL
3/4 teaspoon	4 mL
1 teaspoon	5 mL
1 tablespoon	15 mL
1/4 cup	59 mL
1/2 cup	118 mL
3/4 cup	177 mL
1 cup	235 mL
2 cups	475 mL
3 cups	700 mL
4 cups	1 L

VOLUME EQUIVALENTS(LIQUID)

US STANDARD	US STANDARD (OUNCES)	METRIC (APPROXIMATE)
2 tablespoons	1 fl.oz.	30 mL
1/4 cup	2 fl.oz.	60 mL
1/2 cup	4 fl.oz.	120 mL
1 cup	8 fl.oz.	240 mL
1 1/2 cup	12 fl.oz.	355 mL
2 cups or 1 pint	16 fl.oz.	475 mL
4 cups or 1 quart	32 fl.oz.	1 L
1 gallon	128 fl.oz.	4 L

TEMPERATURES EQUIVALENTS

FAHRENHEIT(F)	CELSIUS(C) (APPROXIMATE)
225 °F	107 °C
250 °F	120 °C
275 °F	135 °C
300 °F	150 °C
325 °F	160 °C
350 °F	180 °C
375 °F	190 °C
400 °F	205 °C
425 °F	220 °C
450 °F	235 °C
475 °F	245 °C
500 °F	260 °C

WEIGHT EQUIVALENTS

US STANDARD	METRIC (APPROXIMATE)
1 ounce	28 g
2 ounces	57 g
5 ounces	142 g
10 ounces	284 g
15 ounces	425 g
16 ounces (1 pound)	455 g
1.5 pounds	680 g
2 pounds	907 g

Chapter 15.
AIR FRYER COOKING CHART

Beef

Item	Temp (°F)	Time (mins)	Item	Temp (°F)	Time (mins)
Beef Eye Round Roast (4 lbs.)	400 °F	45 to 55	Meatballs (1-inch)	370 °F	7
Burger Patty (4 oz.)	370 °F	16 to 20	Meatballs (3-inch)	380 °F	10
Filet Mignon (8 oz.)	400 °F	18	Ribeye, bone-in (1-inch, 8 oz)	400 °F	10 to 15
Flank Steak (1.5 lbs.)	400 °F	12	Sirloin steaks (1-inch, 12 oz)	400 °F	9 to 14
Flank Steak (2 lbs.)	400 °F	20 to 28			

Chicken

Item	Temp (°F)	Time (mins)	Item	Temp (°F)	Time (mins)
Breasts, bone in (1 ¼ lb.)	370 °F	25	Legs, bone-in (1 ¾ lb.)	380 °F	30
Breasts, boneless (4 oz)	380 °F	12	Thighs, boneless (1 ½ lb.)	380 °F	18 to 20
Drumsticks (2 ½ lb.)	370 °F	20	Wings (2 lb.)	400 °F	12
Game Hen (halved 2 lb.)	390 °F	20	Whole Chicken	360 °F	75
Thighs, bone-in (2 lb.)	380 °F	22	Tenders	360 °F	8 to 10

Pork & Lamb

Item	Temp (°F)	Time (mins)	Item	Temp (°F)	Time (mins)
Bacon (regular)	400 °F	5 to 7	Pork Tenderloin	370 °F	15
Bacon (thick cut)	400 °F	6 to 10	Sausages	380 °F	15
Pork Loin (2 lb.)	360 °F	55	Lamb Loin Chops (1-inch thick)	400 °F	8 to 12
Pork Chops, bone in (1-inch, 6.5 oz)	400 °F	12	Rack of Lamb (1.5 – 2 lb.)	380 °F	22

Fish & Seafood

Item	Temp (°F)	Time (mins)	Item	Temp (°F)	Time (mins)
Calamari (8 oz)	400 °F	4	Tuna Steak	400 °F	7 to 10
Fish Fillet (1-inch, 8 oz)	400 °F	10	Scallops	400 °F	5 to 7
Salmon, fillet (6 oz)	380 °F	12	Shrimp	400 °F	5
Swordfish steak	400 °F	10			

Vegetables

INGREDIENT	AMOUNT	PREPARATION	OIL	TEMP	COOK TIME
Asparagus	2 bunches	Cut in half, trim stems	2 Tbsp	420°F	12-15 mins
Beets	1½ lbs	Peel, cut in ½-inch cubes	1Tbsp	390°F	28-30 mins
Bell peppers (for roasting)	4 peppers	Cut in quarters, remove seeds	1Tbsp	400°F	15-20 mins
Broccoli	1 large head	Cut in 1-2-inch florets	1Tbsp	400°F	15-20 mins
Brussels sprouts	1lb	Cut in half, remove stems	1Tbsp	425°F	15-20 mins
Carrots	1lb	Peel, cut in ¼-inch rounds	1 Tbsp	425°F	10-15 mins
Cauliflower	1 head	Cut in 1-2-inch florets	2 Tbsp	400°F	20-22 mins
Corn on the cob	7 ears	Whole ears, remove husks	1 Tbps	400°F	14-17 mins
Green beans	1 bag (12 oz)	Trim	1 Tbps	420°F	18-20 mins
Kale (for chips)	4 oz	Tear into pieces,remove stems	None	325°F	5-8 mins
Mushrooms	16 oz	Rinse, slice thinly	1 Tbps	390°F	25-30 mins
Potatoes, russet	1½ lbs	Cut in 1-inch wedges	1 Tbps	390°F	25-30 mins
Potatoes, russet	1lb	Hand-cut fries, soak 30 mins in cold water, then pat dry	½ -3 Tbps	400°F	25-28 mins
Potatoes, sweet	1lb	Hand-cut fries, soak 30 mins in cold water, then pat dry	1 Tbps	400°F	25-28 mins
Zucchini	1lb	Cut in eighths lengthwise, then cut in half	1 Tbps	400°F	15-20 mins

CONCLUSION

Using an Air Fryer can be hard at first. If you follow our tips and tricks in this book, you will cook like a pro in no time! We've included a variety of recipes in this book, so you'll never run out of gas while attempting to prepare your favorite foods again! Be sure to read the whole book to ensure that you understand anything.

There's something about air fryers. When you think about it, they're kind of like a meal in a bit, without the hassle of actually cooking. Simply grab a slice of bread or your favorite dish (or even a sandwich!), put it in the air fryer oven, and wait for it to cook.

Air-fryers are convenient because they can be used at all hours. You can use them for cooking your favorite dish for dinner while you're getting ready or a mid-day snack. You can even use them for cooking large meals such as breakfast foods or ethnic dishes overnight and saving yourself from having to clean up after dinner.

When you're using an air fryer, though, be careful about what foods you use. Some foods are difficult or impossible to fry when using an air fryer, so avoid using certain ingredients such as breaded chicken and pancakes with syrup or butter. There may be some other things you want to avoid, too, so be sure to check out our article on the Diabetic Air Fryer Cookbook.

The Diabetic Air Fryer Cookbook provides a complete guide to using your air fryer for the first time.

This cookbook is designed to teach you some of the basics about how to use your air fryer, allowing you to enjoy all of its great features. We start with a short list of rules and tips that will help you make sure you are using your air-fryer correctly.

On Diabetic Air-Fryer Cookbook, we provide a full selection of accessories to help you use your air fryer more effectively. We provide an extensive selection of tools to repair your air fryer and make sure it is in peak condition and lasts as long as possible.

After reading our cookbook, you'll find that we've covered all the bases when it comes to using your Diabetic Air Fryer Cookbook. You'll be able to cook healthy food every time with little effort and save money in the process! Make healthier choices without sacrifice from using this innovative and easy-to-use appliance!

One of the coolest ways to cook healthy food in a microwave is to use the air-frying method. It involves cooking with steam, without oil or fats. This means that your kitchen will be free from a "fried" smell, and you can have a healthier diet.

This cookbook's content will help you learn exactly how to do this by following step-by-step directions that will be written for you without confusing words or often used terms. We will teach you how to prepare and cook delicious and nutritious dishes quickly and easily when using an Air Fryer.

Using this method, you will be able to prepare them in under 30 minutes without storing or freezing the ingredients because the foods are not fried at all.

It is just one of the key things that you can get from this book. Along with the "how-to" instructions, you will also receive helpful tips and tricks to help you when cooking with an Air Fryer.

Printed in Great Britain
by Amazon

11469444R00054